A Text Book

PHARMACEUTICAL QUALITY ASSURANCE

As Per PCI Regulations

THIRD YEAR B. PHARM.
Semester VI

Anusuya R. Kashi
Assistant Professor,
Vivekananda College of Pharmacy,
Dr. Raj Kumar Road, Rajajinagar 2nd Stage,
Bengaluru – 560 055, Karnataka, India

Bindu Sukumaran
Assistant Professor,
Vivekananda College of Pharmacy,
Dr. Raj Kumar Road, Rajajinagar 2nd Stage,
Bengaluru – 560 055, Karnataka, India

Venna P.
Assistant Profesor and Vice Principal,
Vivekananda College of Pharmacy,
Dr. Raj Kumar Road, Rajajinagar 2nd Stage,
Bengaluru – 560 055, Karnataka, India

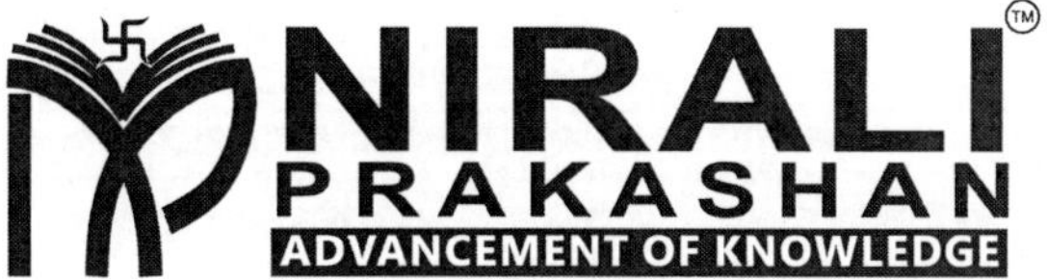

N4088

Pharmaceutical Quality Assurance   **ISBN 978-93-89825-24-4**

First Edition   :   January 2020

©   :   Authors

Published By :
NIRALI PRAKASHAN
Abhyudaya Pragati, 1312, Shivaji Nagar,
Off J.M. Road, PUNE – 411005
Tel - (020) 25512336/37/39, Fax - (020) 25511379
Email : niralipune@pragationline.com

➢ **DISTRIBUTION CENTRES**

PUNE

Nirali Prakashan : 119, Budhwar Peth, Jogeshwari Mandir Lane, Pune 411002, Maharashtra
(For orders within Pune)   Tel : (020) 2445 2044, Fax : (020) 2445 1538; Mobile : 9657703145
Email : niralilocal@pragationline.com

Nirali Prakashan : S. No. 28/27, Dhayari, Near Asian College Pune 411041
(For orders outside Pune)   Tel : (020) 24690204 Fax : (020) 24690316; Mobile : 9657703143
Email : bookorder@pragationline.com

MUMBAI

Nirali Prakashan : 385, S.V.P. Road, Rasdhara Co-op. Hsg. Society Ltd.,
Girgaum, Mumbai 400004, Maharashtra; Mobile : 9320129587
Tel : (022) 2385 6339 / 2386 9976, Fax : (022) 2386 9976
Email : niralimumbai@pragationline.com

➢ **DISTRIBUTION BRANCHES**

JALGAON

Nirali Prakashan : 34, V. V. Golani Market, Navi Peth, Jalgaon 425001, Maharashtra,
Tel : (0257) 222 0395, Mob : 94234 91860; Email : niralijalgaon@pragationline.com

KOLHAPUR

Nirali Prakashan : New Mahadvar Road, Kedar Plaza, 1st Floor Opp. IDBI Bank, Kolhapur 416 012
Maharashtra. Mob : 9850046155; Email : niralikolhapur@pragationline.com

NAGPUR

Nirali Prakashan : Above Maratha Mandir, Shop No. 3, First Floor,
Rani Jhanshi Square, Sitabuldi, Nagpur 440012, Maharashtra
Tel : (0712) 254 7129; Email : pratibhabookdistributors@gmail.com

DELHI

Nirali Prakashan : 4593/15, Basement, Agarwal Lane, Ansari Road, Daryaganj
Near Times of India Building, New Delhi 110002 Mob : 08505972553
Email : niralidelhi@pragationline.com

BENGALURU

Nirali Prakashan : Maitri Ground Floor, Jaya Apartments, No. 99, 6th Cross, 6th Main,
Malleswaram, Bengaluru 560003, Karnataka; Mob : 9449043034
Email: niralibangalore@pragationline.com

Other Branches : Hyderabad, Chennai

niralipune@pragationline.com | www.pragationline.com

Also find us on f www.facebook.com/niralibooks

Preface

In a welcome move, the Pharmacy Council of India has recently re-structured the syllabus of the Bachelor of Pharmacy course. In the effort to make the content more relevant to the practice of pharmacy in its current form, we now find new, important subjects introduced, and Pharmaceutical Quality Assurance is one of them.

While quality is the single-most important requirement for any product, it becomes even more critical in the pharmaceutical industry where patients rely on medicines to cure, prevent and mitigate diseases. From the times when mere quality control testing was sufficient to approve products as fit for use, we have now progressed to the realization that quality must be built into drug products from the very initial design phase. Quality assurance (QA) comprises the sum total of all that goes into ensuring that products manufactured are of the intended quality that makes them fit for use. Understanding the several different aspects of QA is therefore a vital first step in working towards attaining desired quality products.

It gives us great pleasure to present this Textbook of Pharmaceutical Quality Assurance to the students of the B. Pharm. course. It has been our endeavour to make the content student-friendly and towards this end, we have included objectives at the beginning and review questions at the end of each chapter. While we have tried to verify all details provided in this book, it is quite possible that some information may need greater clarity or amendment – if you, the readers, notice any errors or scope for improvement, we will be most obliged to receive your feedback and suggestions.

For teachers, explaining concepts in a classroom is very easy; writing the same content in a lucid style that holds students' attention is definitely more challenging. We thank our family and friends for their encouragement in achieving this milestone. We express special thanks to Mr. R. E. Narayana, our senior librarian in the Vivekananda College of Pharmacy who put us in touch with Mr. Ramakrishna of Nirali Prakashan and sowed the initial idea of writing this textbook. Their encouragement has been instrumental in guiding our efforts. It has also been a pleasure to work with Ms. Roshan Khan, Co-ordinator of Pharmacy Department of Nirali Prakashan.

We are grateful to the management of the Janatha Education Society for their support to this venture. We are deeply grateful to our college Principal, Dr. D. Narasimha Reddy, for his constant support and guidance.

We also take this opportunity to thank Ms. Vasundhara Rama Iyengar for her help in structuring the content of this textbook. With close to 30 years of service in the pharmaceutical industry, having served as the Quality Head in reputed pharmaceutical companies such as AstraZeneca Pharma India Limited and GlaxoSmithKline Pharmaceuticals Limited, her suggestions have added immensely to the value of our work.

With a sense of deep gratitude to the Almighty for blessing us with the necessary skills and resources, we offer this book to B. Pharm. students from all over the country. We trust this book will enable them to understand the multiple aspects of QA in the pharma industry. We also hope it will kindle a sense of pride in being part of the profession of Pharmacy that contributes so greatly to human welfare.

Anusuya R. Kashi
Bindu Sukumaran
Veena P.

Syllabus

UNIT I   **(10 Hours)**

Quality Assurance and Quality Management Concepts: Definition and Concept of Quality Control, Quality Assurance and GMP.

Total Quality Management (TQM): Definition, elements, philosophies.

ICH Guidelines: Purpose, Participants, Process of Harmonization, Brief Overview of QSEM, with special emphasis on Q-series guidelines, ICH stability testing guidelines.

Quality by design (QbD): Definition, overview, elements of QbD program, tools.

ISO 9000 & ISO14000: Overview, Benefits, Elements, steps for registration.

NABL accreditation: Principles and Procedures.

UNIT II   **(10 Hours)**

Organization and Personnel: Personnel responsibilities, Training, Hygiene and Personal records.

Premises: Design, Construction and plant layout, Maintenance, Sanitation, environmental control, utilities and maintenance of sterile areas, Control of contamination.

Equipments and Raw Materials: Equipment selection, Purchase specifications, Maintenance, Purchase specifications and maintenance of stores for raw materials.

UNIT III   **(10 Hours)**

Quality Control: Quality control test for containers, Rubber closures and secondary packing materials.

Good Laboratory Practices: General Provisions, Organization and Personnel, Facilities, Equipment, Testing Facilities Operation, Test and Control Articles, Protocol for Conduct of a Non-clinical Laboratory Study, Records and Reports, Disqualification of Testing Facilities.

UNIT IV   **(08 Hours)**

Complaints: Complaints and evaluation of complaints, Handling of return good, recalling and waste disposal.

Document Maintenance in Pharmaceutical Industry: Batch Formula Record, Master Formula, Record, SOP, Quality audit, Quality Review and Quality documentation, Reports and documents, Distribution records.

UNIT V   **(07 Hours)**

Calibration and Validation: Introduction, definition and general principles of calibration, Qualification and validation, Importance and scope of validation, Types of validation, Validation master plan. Calibration of pH meter, Qualification of UV-Visible spectrophotometer, General Principles of Analytical method Validation.

Warehousing: Good warehousing practice, materials management

✍ ✍ ✍

Contents

UNIT - I

1. Quality Assurance and Quality Management Concept — 1.1 - 1.8
1.1 History of Drug Regulations — 1.1
1.2 The Regulatory Drug Approval Process — 1.4
1.3 Quality Assurance — 1.5
    1.3.1 Objectives of Quality Assurance — 1.5
1.4 Current Good Manufacturing Practices (cGMP) — 1.6
1.5 Quality Control — 1.7
    1.5.1 Objectives of Quality Control — 1.7
• Review Questions — 1.8

2. Total Quality Management — 2.1 - 2.6
2.1 Evolution of Quality Management — 2.1
2.2 Definition of TQM — 2.2
2.3 Key Elements of TQM — 2.3
2.4 Philosophies of TQM — 2.4
2.5 TQM in Drug Industry — 2.5
    2.5.1 Quality by Design — 2.5
• Review Questions — 2.6

3. International Conference on Harmonization (ICH) — 3.1 - 3.8
3.1 ICH and its Purpose — 3.1
3.2 History of ICH — 3.2
3.3 Process of Harmonization — 3.3
3.4 ICH Guidelines: Quality, Safety, Efficacy, Multidisciplinary (QSEM) — 3.4
3.5 Quality Guidelines — 3.5
3.6 ICH Guidelines for Stability — 3.6
    3.6.1 Types of Stability Testing — 3.7
    3.6.2 Stability Testing Protocol — 3.7
    3.6.3 Overview of ICH Stability Guidelines Contents — 3.7
• Review Questions — 3.8

4. Pharmaceutical Quality by Design — 4.1 - 4.8
4.1 Definition — 4.2
4.2 Overview — 4.2
4.3 Elements of QbD — 4.3
4.4 Quality by Design Tools — 4.6
    4.4.1 Prior Knowledge — 4.6
    4.4.2 Risk Assessment — 4.7
    4.4.3 Design of Experiments — 4.7
    4.4.4 Process Analytical Technology (PAT) — 4.7
• Review Questions — 4.8

5. Introduction to ISO 9000 and ISO 14000 — 5.1 - 5.5
5.1 History of ISO — 5.1
5.2 Overview of ISO — 5.1
5.3 Aim of ISO International Standards — 5.2
5.4 ISO 9000 Family — 5.2
    5.4.1 Criteria to get ISO 9001 Certification — 5.3
    5.4.2 Benefits of ISO 9001 Certification — 5.3
5.5 ISO 14000 — 5.4
    5.5.1 Aim of ISO 14000 Standards — 5.4
    5.5.2 Benefits of ISO 14000 — 5.5
• Review Questions — 5.5

6. NABL Accredition   **6.1 - 6.5**
6.1   Introduction   6.1
•   Review Questions   6.5

UNIT - II

7. Organization and Personnel   **7.1 - 7.4**
7.1   Organization   7.1
7.2   Responsibilities of QC Unit   7.2
7.3   Personnel Responsibilities   7.2
7.4   Personnel Qualifications   7.3
7.5   Key Personnel   7.3
7.6   Personnel Training   7.3
7.7   Personnel Health and Hygiene   7.4
•   Review Questions   7.4

8. Premises - Design, Construction Layout and Maintenance   **8.1 - 8.8**
8.1   Location   8.1
8.2   Design and Construction   8.2
8.3   Utilities   8.2
8.4   Sanitation   8.3
    8.4.1   Sanitation of Sterile Areas   8.3
8.5   Environmental Control   8.3
8.6   Contamination   8.4
8.7   Cross Contamination   8.5
    8.7.1   Measures to Prevent/ Reduce Cross-contamination   8.6
    8.7.2   Preventing Dust Migration in Non-dedicated Facilities   8.6
    8.7.3   Air Containment   8.6
    8.7.4   Airlocks   8.7
8.8   Additional Considerations Regarding Premises   8.7
    8.8.1   Storage Areas   8.7
    8.8.2   Production Areas   8.8
    8.8.3   Quality Control (QC) Laboratory Areas   8.8
•   Review Questions   8.8

9. Equipments and Raw Materials   **9.1 - 9.6**
9.1   Equipments   9.1
    9.1.1   Design and Construction   9.1
    9.1.2   Location   9.2
    9.1.3   Installation   9.2
    9.1.4   Cleaning and Maintenance   9.2
    9.1.5   Qualification and Calibration   9.2
    9.1.6   Documentation   9.3
    9.1.7   Purchase Specifications for Equipment   9.3
9.2   Raw Material   9.4
    9.2.1   Purchase of Materials   9.4
    9.2.3   Receiving, handling and storage of materials   9.4
    9.2.4   Sampling   9.5
    9.2.5   Testing of Samples   9.5
    9.2.6   Approval/Rejection of Materials   9.5
    9.2.7   Labeling   9.5
    9.2.8   Using Approved Materials   9.5
    9.2.9   Handling Rejected Materials   9.6
    9.2.10   Containers and Closures   9.6
•   Review Questions   9.6

UNIT - III

10. Quality Control																					**10.1 - 10.20**

10.1	Definition	10.1
	10.1.1 WHO	10.1
	10.1.2 Schedule M	10.2
10.2	Scope of QC	10.2
10.3	Organization of QC	10.2
10.4	Responsibilities of QC	10.2
10.5	Sampling	10.3
10.6	Testing and Analysis	10.3
10.7	Product Assessment	10.3
10.8	Reference Samples/Retained Samples	10.4
10.9	Out Of Specifications (OOS) Results	10.4
10.11	Drug Packaging	10.6
10.12	Functions of Packaging	10.6
10.13	Classification of Pharmaceutical Packaging	10.6
10.14	Quality Control of Packaging Materials	10.6
10.15	Parameters Tested	10.7
10.16	Tests on Containers as Per Indian Pharmacopoeia	10.9
	10.16.1 Tests on Glass Containers	10.9
	10.16.2 Metal Containers for Eye Ointments	10.12
	10.16.3 Plastic Containers and Closures	10.13
	10.16.4 Rubber Closures for Parenteral Product Containers	10.16
10.17	Tests for Paper and Boards	10.17
	10.17.1 Dimensions	10.17
	10.17.2 Thickness	10.17
	10.17.3 Grammage	10.17
	10.17.4 pH of Surface	10.18
	10.17.5 pH of Extract	10.18
	10.17.6 Alkalinity	10.18
	10.17.7 Moisture Content	10.18
	10.17.8 Ash Content	10.18
	10.17.9 Cobb Test	10.18
	10.17.10 Other Tests for Paper/Board/Cartons	10.19
•	Review Questions	10.20

11. Good Laboratory Practices for Non-Clinical Laboratories					**11.1 - 11.10**

11.1	Definition of GLP	11.2
11.2	Scope of GLP	11.2
11.3	Personnel	11.2
11.4	Organization and Management of Test Facility	11.3
	11.4.1 Study Director	11.3
	11.4.2 Systems	11.3
	11.4.3 Management	11.3
	11.4.4 QA Unit	11.3
11.5	Facilities	11.4
	11.5.1 Animal Care Facilities	11.4
	11.5.2 Animal Supply Facilities	11.4
	11.5.3 Test and Control Handling Facilities	11.4
	11.5.4 Laboratory Operation Areas	11.4
	11.5.5 Specimen and Data Storage Facilities	11.4

11.6	Equipment		11.4
	11.6.1	Design and Location	11.4
	11.6.2	Calibration and Maintenance	11.4
11.7	Testing Facilities Operation		11.5
	11.7.1	Standard Operating Procedures (SOPs)	11.5
	11.7.2	Solutions and Reagents	11.5
	11.7.3	Animal Care	11.5
	11.7.4	Characterization of Test and Control Articles	11.6
	11.7.5	Handling of Control and Test Articles	11.6
	11.7.6	Article-carrier Mixtures	11.6
11.8	Protocol for and Conduct of Non-clinical Laboratory Study		11.6
	11.8.1	Protocol	11.6
	11.8.2	Conduct of the Study	11.7
11.9	Records and Reports		11.7
	11.9.1	Reporting Study Results	11.7
	11.9.2	Data and Records Storage and Retrieval	11.8
	11.9.3	Retaining Records	11.8
11.10	Disqualification of Testing Facilities		11.9
	11.10.1	Purpose	11.9
	11.10.2	Disqualification Grounds	11.9
	11.10.3	Final Disqualification Order	11.9
	11.10.4	Actions Following Disqualification	11.9
	11.10.5	Public Disclosure of Disqualification	11.10
	11.10.6	Termination or Suspension of Testing Facility by Sponsor	11.10
	11.10.7	Reinstatement of a Disqualified Testing Facility	11.10
•	Review Questions		11.10

UNIT - IV

12. Complaint, Recalls and Waste Disposal   12.1 - 12.12

12.1	Steps in Complaint Handling		12.2
	12.1.1	Receiving the Complaint	12.2
	12.1.2	Technical Examination and Investigation of the Complaint	12.2
	12.1.3	Document-Based Investigation	12.3
	12.1.4	Laboratory Analysis	12.3
	12.1.5	Corrective Measures and Giving Feedback to Complainant	12.3
	12.1.6	Trend Analysis	12.4
12.2	Drug Recalls		12.4
	12.2.1	Types of Recall	12.5
	12.2.2	Recall is Different from Withdrawal	12.5
	12.2.3	Reasons for Product Recall	12.6
	12.2.4	Classification of Recall	12.6
	12.2.5	Mock Recall	12.7
	12.2.6	Product Recall System	12.8
12.3	Handling Returned Goods		12.9
12.4	Waste Disposal		12.9
	12.4.1	Types of Waste	12.10
	12.4.2	Disposal of Pharmaceutical Waste	12.10
	12.4.3	Effluent Treatment of Pharmaceutical Waste	12.12
•	Review Questions		12.12

13. Documentation in Pharmaceutical Industry   13.1 - 13.14

13.1	Importance of Documentation in Pharmaceutical Industry	13.2
13.2	Good Documentation Practices	13.2
13.3	Types of Documents	13.4

13.4	Master Formula Record (MFR)	13.5
13.5	Batch Manufacturing Record (BMR)	13.6
13.6	Standard Operating Procedure (SOP)	13.7
13.7	Quality Review	13.10
13.8	Quality Audits	13.11
13.9	Quality Documentation	13.12
13.10	Distribution Records	13.13
•	Review Questions	13.13

UNIT - V

14. Calibration and Validation 14.1 - 14.18

14.1	Calibration	14.1
	14.1.1 Definition	14.2
	14.1.2 Objectives of Calibration	14.2
	14.1.3 Significance of Calibration	14.2
	14.1.4 Frequency of Calibration	14.3
	14.1.5 Calibration Methods	14.3
14.2	Qualification	14.3
	14.2.1 Definition	14.4
	14.2.2 Phases of Qualification	14.4
	14.2.3 Considerations While Doing Qualification	14.5
	14.2.4 Requalification	14.5
	14.2.5 Factory Acceptance Test and Site Acceptance Test	14.5
14.3	Validation	14.6
	14.3.1 History of Validation	14.6
	14.3.2 Definition	14.6
	14.3.3 Scope of Validation	14.7
	14.3.4 Advantages of Validation	14.7
	14.3.5 Types of Validation	14.8
	14.3.6 Revalidation	14.10
	14.3.7 Validation Master Plan	14.11
	14.3.8 Analytical Method Validation	14.13
•	Review Questions	14.18

15. Good Warehousing Practice and Materials Management 15.1 - 15.6

15.1	Personnel	15.1
15.2	Premises and Facilities	15.2
	15.2.1 Storage Areas	15.2
	15.2.2 Storage Conditions	15.3
15.3	Storage Requirements	15.3
	15.3.1 Documentation	15.3
	15.3.2 Labelling and Containers	15.4
	15.3.3 Receiving Incoming Materials	15.4
	15.3.4 Stock Rotation and Control	15.5
	15.3.5 Control of Obsolete and Outdated Products	15.5
15.4	Returned Goods	15.5
15.5	Dispatch and Transportation of Goods	15.5
15.6	Product Recall	15.6
•	Review Questions	15.6
References		**R.1 - R.4**

Chapter ... 1

QUALITY ASSURANCE AND QUALITY MANAGEMENT CONCEPT

Objectives:

Upon completion of this section, the student should be able to

- Describe the major events that led to the development of quality concepts in the pharmaceutical industry.
- List the important pharmaceutical regulatory bodies across the world.
- Understand the drug approval process.
- Define the terms 'Quality Assurance' and 'Quality Control' and their objectives.
- Differentiate between Quality Assurance and Quality Control.
- Define the term Good Manufacturing Practices (GMPs).
- Explain the areas covered under current Good Manufacturing Practices (cGMPs).

Introduction

Quality is an important requirement for products in any industry because it directly determines the profits realized from their sale. However, in the pharmaceutical industry, there is yet another important reason why quality products are necessary. In fact, this is one of the major reasons why this industry is so highly regulated – because any errors in the manufacturing process can lead to dangerous and even fatal results for the patients consuming the products. Therefore, it is vital that pharmaceutical products must be manufactured to meet stringent regulatory standards.

1.1 HISTORY OF DRUG REGULATIONS

In the field of drug products, it is the United States of America that has always been at the forefront of developing the necessary regulatory guidelines, and the trend continues to this day. Much of the history of drug regulations therefore cover events in the US.

In the olden days, medicines were prepared mainly in the form of elixirs, ointments and pills, and sold by the person making them. These medicine containers were labeled with nothing much beyond the name of the product they contained, and the troubles they promised to cure. Later, as science and technology advanced, some small family businesses began manufacturing other products like vaccines and anti-toxins too, but there was almost no control over these operations.

In 1902, a mishap occurred to focus attention on the dangers of such manufacturing. Twelve children died after being administered an antitoxin for diphtheria and it was found that the product had been contaminated with live tetanus bacilli. In response to strong protests from the public, the United States Congress passed the Biologics Control Act. Under this Act, the manufacturers and sellers of such biological products had to test their products for strength and purity; they also had to undergo regular inspections by the health authorities.

In 1906, the US Congress passed the Pure Food and Drug Act. This made it illegal for people to sell adulterated/contaminated food or meat. Medicines were now required to have labels that stated the true facts about their contents, without any false information or promising magical cures. Out of this Act was born one of the world's first government regulatory bodies, which we now known as the United States Food and Drug Administration (USFDA).

This body was conferred the authority to seize illegal drugs and foods. Any dangerous ingredients in medicines now had to be labeled, and the labeling had to be true and accurate.

In 1935, 107 people, a majority of them children, died after consuming oral sulfanilamide elixir. An investigation showed that this product had been made using a solvent called diethylene glycol which is a poisonous solvent! The public was incensed and demanded stricter laws.

In response, the US Congress passed the Federal Food, Drug and Cosmetic Act of 1938. For the first time in the history of drug manufacturing, it became necessary for companies to prove that the products made by them were safe, before allowing them into the market. This Act also made factory inspections mandatory, set down standards for food products, and made penalties and criminal proceedings more stringent.

In 1941, yet another tragedy occurred in which close to 300 people died. The cause was Sulfathiazole tablets had got contaminated with a sedative Phenobarbital. This led to significant changes in the regulations controlling manufacturing and quality control requirements for drugs. The Public Health Services (PHS) Act that was passed in 1944 further expanded the scope of regulations to biological products.

The process of certification of batches by the FDA began during the time of World War II. Manufacturers of insulin, penicillin and other antibiotics would submit samples to the FDA from each lot they made and get permission for the release of these products.

In 1955, days after a mass polio vaccination drive began using the newly developed Salk polio vaccine, it had to be abandoned. The reason was children who received the vaccine (from batches made by Cutter Laboratories) were found to have developed the disease.

An investigation showed that there had been a failure in the process of inactivating the live polio virus, and this had gone undetected! This incident was widely discussed internationally and brought home the need for even more control over the safety standards of vaccines. The worst was yet to come, though.

In 1957, a pharmaceutical company in Germany called Chemie Grunenthal GmbH developed the world's first non-barbiturate anti-convulsant drug called as Thalidomide. It was found to also have a sedative effect and doctors began prescribing it as a tranquilizer.

Thalidomide was sold over-the-counter based only on the claims of its manufacturer. Laboratory studies on animals showed it was practically impossible to reach a LD50 dose. (LD50 is the lethal dose which causes death in 50% of the animals tested.) So the company advertised it as totally safe even for mother-and-child. This "wonder drug" became hugely popular and was marketed to 46 countries across the world.

Around 1960, an Australian obstetrician McBride noticed that the drug also helped to reduce the morning sickness associated with pregnancy. He began recommending it to his pregnant patients, and through word-of-mouth reports in the medical fraternity, this practice, too spread across the world. Only in the USA, the drug had not been approved for use by the FDA's drug examiner named Frances Kelsey. (Years later, she was conferred with awards for the service she had rendered to the American public through this act.)

However, by 1961, McBride began noticing a severe birth defect called phocomelia in babies delivered by his patients who had taken Thalidomide. Phocomelia is the condition where a baby has no limbs, or shortened or flipper-like limbs. A newspaper in Germany reported that close to 161 babies had been thus adversely affected by the drug, and the distribution of Thalidomide in Germany was stopped, with other countries following suit. By 1962, after at least 10,000 cases of deformed infants had been born, Thalidomide was finally completely banned.

This shocking tragedy was the catalyst for putting in place a more rigorous drug approval and quality monitoring system developed by the USFDA. Companies were now required to test both efficacy and safety of their drugs. Drugs had to be tested on animals before they could be tried on humans. Clinical trial regulations became more stringent and the drug investigators were made responsible for supervising the drugs being studied. In other words, companies now had to obtain consent from the regulatory authorities before testing a drug and had to prove the drug's safety and efficacy before manufacturing it and taking it to the market.

It was only in 1963 that the USFDA published the first ever set of Good Manufacturing Practices (GMP) for finished pharmaceuticals.

Today, GMP or current Good Manufacturing Practices (cGMP), as it is now known, is the very backbone of ensuring the quality, safety and efficacy of drug products. Every country has regulatory bodies to oversee the drug development, manufacturing and distribution process. These bodies lay down cGMP guidelines that ensure all processes right from procuring materials to drug manufacturing to their distribution occurs under the most stringent of controls.

Global Regulatory Bodies

Country	Regulatory body
USA	Food & Drug Administration (FDA)
Japan	Ministry of Health Labour and Welfare
Australia	Therapeutic Goods Administration (TGA)
UK	Medicines and Healthcare products Regulatory Agency (MHRA)
South Africa	Medicine Control Council (MCC)
India	Central Drugs Standard Control Organization (CDSCO)
China	State Food and Drug Administration

1.2 THE REGULATORY DRUG APPROVAL PROCESS

Drug development is a complex process and the transition of a molecule from the laboratory bench to the patient's bedside is a long and arduous journey that can take anywhere from 10 – 15 years at the very least.

A drug company first chooses a biochemical mechanism that is the basis of some disease, and begins screening molecules to overcome that condition. Through the use of proteomics, functional genomics and other screening methods, a few lead molecules that show promise are chosen for characterization.

Characterization involves the study of the molecule's shape, size, strengths, bioactivity, weaknesses, toxicity, bioavailability and the possible mechanism of its action. Next, work commences on formulating the molecule into a suitable dosage form for administration. This involves a study of the drug's stability to heat, light, and within the formulation itself.

This stage is followed by an investigation of the pharmacokinetics of the drug and ADME (Absorption/Distribution/Metabolism/Excretion) studies to get information that also helps to improve the formulation.

Next come the pre-clinical toxicology tests for acute toxicity, repeated dose toxicity, and genetic and, reproductive toxicity, carcinogenicity etc. Armed with results from all these tests, the company files an Investigative New Drug Application (INDA) with the FDA, who scrutinizes the application and if satisfied, gives the green signal for the clinical trials to begin.

Clinical research trials are held in three phases – the first is to test the safety of the drug in healthy human volunteers; the second phase is run with 100 – 250 patients who suffer from the disease, and the third phase is performed on even larger groups of patients in multi-center trials. By this stage, if the molecule still proves to be safe and effective, the company files the New Drug Application with the FDA. Following a regulatory review of this, the FDA takes the decision about approving or not approving the drug for manufacture. Approved drugs then enter into the fourth phase of clinical research which is the post-marketing surveillance study that is closely monitored by the FDA.

From a study of this entire process, it is quite clear that drug development is a time-consuming and costly affair. For every 5000 molecules that enter the process, only about 5 make it to the stage of clinical testing and probably just 1 out of those 5 gets FDA approval.

1.3 QUALITY ASSURANCE

Getting FDA approval is however only the start of yet another equally tough journey. The drug formulation has to transit from the laboratory to the manufacturing floor, which has its own challenges. As obvious from the history of how cGMP came into being, there are many things that can go wrong and it is vital to have sufficient control over all the factors that can influence the quality of the final drug product.

For several years, pharmaceutical companies relied a lot on Quality Control (QC) for adequate testing of the quality of their products. With time, however, as processing operations grew more complex, the realization grew that testing often misses detecting problems because tests are run on randomly selected samples. One cannot hope to "test quality into" products that do not have the quality inherent in them.

This realization led to the development of the concept of Quality Assurance (QA) which seeks to build quality into the products from the very beginning of the process of drug manufacture. By careful planning, training and monitoring QA is a means to control processes right from choosing the right vendor for the starting and packing materials, to the manner in which distribution of finished product takes place. The aim is to cover all the aspects that individually and collectively impact the quality of products.

The World Health Organization (WHO) defines QA as, "The totality of arrangements made with the object of ensuring that pharmaceutical products are of the quality required for their intended use."

1.3.1 Objectives of Quality Assurance

The objectives of QA system in a pharmaceutical industry are to ensure that:

- Product design and development is in accordance with requirements of cGMP, Good Laboratory Practices (for non-clinical developmental studies) and Good Clinical Practices (for clinical studies).
- All operations in production and control steps are specified clearly in writing.
- Managerial responsibility is specified clearly in each job description.
- Correct starting materials and packaging materials are used to manufacture drug products.
- Appropriate controls – such as in-process checks, calibrations and validations – exist to ensure quality of raw materials, intermediate products and finished products.
- Finished products are appropriately checked in accordance with pre-determined procedures.

- Every production batch is certified by authorized persons before it is released for sale and supply.
- There are satisfactory measures adopted to ensure quality of the product which is maintained throughout its shelf life.
- Procedures exist for regular self-inspection or quality audits to assess the effectiveness of the QA system.
- Deviations of any nature are reported, adequately investigated and the results are recorded.
- Changes having an impact on product quality are adopted through a system that calls for approval from management.
- Quality of products is regularly evaluated in order to verify that the process is consistently providing quality products.

1.4 CURRENT GOOD MANUFACTURING PRACTICES (cGMP)

cGMP is the aspect of QA that ensures the consistent production and control of products to meet pre-determined quality standards. The primary aim of cGMP is to reduce two inherent risks involved in pharmaceutical production – mix-ups and cross-contamination. Mix-up refers to the confusion caused by interchange of materials, whereas cross-contamination is unexpected contamination of one batch of product by another product.

cGMP guidelines are prescribed by every country's drug regulatory authority and according to WHO, cGMP requires that :

(a) All manufacturing processes are clearly defined, systematically reviewed in the light of experience, and shown to be capable of consistently manufacturing pharmaceutical products of the required quality that comply with their specifications;

(b) Qualification and validation are performed;

(c) All necessary resources are provided, including:

    (i)   Appropriately qualified and trained personnel;

    (ii) Adequate premises and space;

    (iii) Suitable equipment and services;

    (iv) Appropriate materials, containers and labels;

    (v) Approved procedures and instructions;

    (vi) Suitable storage and transport;

    (vii) Adequate personnel, laboratories and equipment for in-process controls;

(d) Instructions and procedures are written in clear and unambiguous language, specifically applicable to the facilities provided;

(e) Operators are trained to carry out procedures correctly;

(f) Records are made (manually and/or by recording instruments) during manufacture to show that all the steps required by the defined procedures and instructions have in fact been taken and that the quantity and quality of the product are as expected; any significant deviations are fully recorded and investigated;

(g) Records covering manufacture and distribution, which enable the complete history of a batch to be traced, are retained in a comprehensible and accessible form;

(h) The proper storage and distribution of the products minimizes any risk to their quality;

(i) A system is available to recall any batch of product from sale or supply;

(j) Complaints about marketed products are examined; the causes of quality defects are investigated, and appropriate measures taken in respect of the defective products to prevent recurrence.

1.5 QUALITY CONTROL

As per ISO 9000, Quality Control (QC) is defined as, "A part of quality management focused on fulfilling quality requirements."

WHO defines QC as, "The sum of all procedures undertaken to ensure the identity and purity of a particular pharmaceutical."

QC is the part of GMP that deals with developing specifications, sampling input materials, intermediates and finished products; testing them, documenting results, and setting up release procedures to ensure that all relevant testing has been performed and only products with ascertained quality are released for use.

1.5.1 Objectives of Quality Control

The objectives of QC department in a pharmaceutical industry are to ensure that:

- There is a day-to-day control maintained over the quality aspects of drug products.
- Incoming raw materials, in-process goods and finished products are all tested for compliance with predetermined quality specifications.
- Environmental monitoring is performed to make sure products are manufactured, packed and stored under prescribed conditions.
- Instruments are calibrated and working as expected.
- Analytical methods are developed and validated to assure they stay capable of providing results that are accurate and predictable.

Differences between QA and QC

Attribute	QA	QC
Goal	Preventing defects.	Identifying defects.
Focus	Building quality into product from design stage itself.	Testing if quality exists in product after its manufacture.
Work flow	Establish quality management system, continuous monitoring of processes.	Find source of problems in quality.
Type of tool	Managerial.	Corrective.

Given the rapid pace at which the pharmaceutical environment is changing today, companies must adapt to the quality requirements needed to consistently manufacture and deliver products with zero-defects. There can be no compromise on the efficacy, quality and safety attributes of drug products. Developing, manufacturing and selling a quality product is a collective responsibility of everyone in an organization. This calls for an integrated approach that includes building quality into a product by design, development of quality management systems that are strictly monitored and focusing on continual improvement to meet consumers' health requirements.

REVIEW QUESTIONS

1. Name the important regulatory bodies that govern the pharmaceutical industry.
2. Discuss how the cGMPs were developed by the USFDA.
3. Explain the steps involved in developing a drug from initial discovery to final marketing of the formulation.
4. Define the terms QA and QC and explain the differences between them.
5. Describe the functions of QA and QC in a pharmaceutical company.
6. What is cGMP? Highlight the important areas covered under cGMP guidelines.

✍ ✍ ✍

*Chapter ...***2**

TOTAL QUALITY MANAGEMENT

Objectives:

Upon completion of this section, the student should be able to

- Explain the major stages in the quality movement.
- Define 'Total Quality Management' (TQM).
- List and explain the key elements of TQM.
- List the philosophies and tools of TQM.
- Explain the concept of quality in the pharmaceutical industry.

Introduction

Quality is a term that is widely used when talking about how good or poor a product or service is. However, defining this term is not so easy. In most cases, it refers to how well the product is able to match the specifications and meet the customer's expectations. ISO defines quality as "The degree to which a set of inherent characteristics fulfills the requirements."

2.1 EVOLUTION OF QUALITY MANAGEMENT

In the early 1900s, businesses were looking for ways to reduce the number of faulty products being produced. In 1911, Frederick W. Taylor published a book titled "The Principles of Scientific Management" which focused on how organizations must use people effectively. He proposed the concept of 'clearly defined tasks' and 'standard conditions' and proposed people be assigned for the purpose of 'inspection' of goods. This led to the birth of the "Inspection Department" and its focus was on preventing defects which in turn, developed into the concept of Quality Control.

During the 1930s, Dr. W. Shewhart developed methods for statistical analysis of production process. Through use of a 'control chart' he showed how variations in manufacturing processes lead to variations in quality of the product. His theory of Statistical Quality Control highlighted the detection and control of problems in quality by testing several samples at different stages of the production process.

During the 1940s, Japanese industry leaders wanted to change the quality of their products which were largely seen as cheap imitations. At their invitation, western quality experts such as W. Edwards Deming, Joseph M. Juran and Armand V. Feigenbaum visited Japan to guide these industries with their quality needs.

Deming taught the Japanese the concepts of statistical analysis and using it for quality control. Juran's teachings focused on the idea of getting managers involved with the quality process. In the early 60s, the Japanese firms came up with 'quality circles' that comprised a voluntary group of workers who met to discuss about improving some aspect of their work and then presented their thoughts to the management. This led to employees feeling more motivated to contribute to the workplace. Gradually, the discussions began to center around improvements that could be made in all organizational areas and not merely the quality of products. This is how the idea of 'Total Quality' originated.

In 1969, Feigenbaum presented a paper at the first international conference on quality control in Tokyo. In it, he used the term 'Total Quality' for the first time. Around the same time, Ishikawa in Japan also came up with the concept of 'Total Quality Control' which differed from the western theory of total quality.

By observing the great strides made by Japan in dealing with quality issues, industry leaders in the West began their own set of quality initiatives in the 1980s and 1990s. These ideas covered a large spectrum of techniques and strategies, and it was all covered by the term 'Total Quality Management' or "TQM."

2.2 DEFINITION OF TQM

Today, TQM has evolved greatly from those initial days, and every day, there is some or the other innovation being added to the term. TQM is defined in several ways, such as:

'TQM is a management system and philosophy that strives towards constant organizational improvement in order to achieve excellence and ensure customer satisfaction and loyalty.'

'TQM is the continued process of detecting/reducing/eliminating errors in manufacturing, streamlining the process of supply chain management, improving customer experience, and ensuring employees are well-trained.'

'TQM is a structured approach to organizational management with a process focused on improving the quality of outputs of an organization, including services and goods, by the constant improvement of its internal practices.'

'TQM is an organizational management philosophy seeking to continuously improve the quality of processes and products.'

Using a set of management and quality tools, TQM approach seeks to increase business even as it reduces loss due to improper practices. Being a highly adaptable concept, it has been widely applied in several industries in the production and service sectors.

The main components of TQM include:

- Focus on consumer
- Analysis of process
- Work in quality teams
- Systematic analysis of problems
- Implement planned changes and evaluate results

- Use data to identify problems and solutions
- Implement changes

TQM focuses on continuous improvement at all levels right from planning up to execution on the shop floor. The main concern is to avoid mistakes and thus, prevent defects in the products. By regular improvement of personnel, equipment, processes and capabilities, it seeks to ensure quality that is consistent. TQM is also based on the main principle that mistakes are often a result of faulty processes and systems and not of individuals per se. By identifying the causes of such mistakes, it is possible to eliminate them through three mechanisms:

- Prevent errors from occurring.
- Where prevention is not possible, early detection to prevent the mistake causing damage down the chain.
- Immediate correction of process if mistakes recur.

2.3 KEY ELEMENTS OF TQM

There are eight key elements on which an organization must focus to implement TQM with success:

(a) Ethics

(b) Integrity

(c) Trust

(d) Training

(e) Teamwork

(f) Leadership

(g) Recognition

(h) Communication

These eight elements are further clubbed into four groups as follows, based on their function:

(a) Group I – Foundation – Ethics, Integrity and Trust

(b) Group II – Building Bricks – Training, Teamwork and Leadership

(c) Group III – Binding Mortar – Communication

(d) Group IV – Roof - Recognition

1. Foundation:

A foundation of ethics, integrity and trust helps to create an open and fair environment that fosters involvement by everyone in the organization. Ethics deals with what is good and bad in a given situation, both at the individual and the organizational levels. Integrity refers to the honesty with which one adheres to facts. When ethics are followed with integrity, it leads to development of trust, the third element of the 'foundation', which creates an environment of cooperativeness.

2. Building Bricks:

Employees need to be trained in performing their duties right and in problem solving. They must also be trained in interacting with others, to do their job better through teamwork. Any team is only as good as its leader, though, and so, there has to be inspirational leadership by someone who understands TQM and is committed to it in daily practice.

3. Binding Mortar:

The link which binds all elements of TQM is communication which refers to a common understanding of the message by both the sender and receiver. Openness in communication between members of an organization, and with vendors, and customers is key to the success of TQM.

4. Roof:

Recognizing the contributions of people in an organization, whether for teams or for individuals, is the final element in TQM. When employees receive recognition, it brings about a leap in their self-esteem and such employees are more motivated which ultimately leads to better productivity and quality of work they do.

2.4 PHILOSOPHIES OF TQM

Several quality experts have given their viewpoints on how to achieve quality. Some of the most important concepts have been summed up in the table below:

Walter A. Shewhart	Understanding variability, concept of statistical control charts
W. Edwards Deming	Management's responsibility for quality, 14 points for quality improvement
Joseph M. Juran	Concept of quality cost, quality trilogy (quality planning, quality control, quality improvement)
Armand E. Feigenbaum	Total quality control
Philip B. Crosby	Concept of zero defects, do it right the first time
Kaoru Ishikawa	Concept of internal customer, quality circles
Genichi Taguchi	Concept of product design quality, developed Taguchi loss function

Advantages of TQM:

- Innovation in processes
- Greater productivity
- Reduced defects in product
- Increased customer satisfaction
- Higher profitability and reduced costs
- Higher employee morale
- Better adaptability to changing market conditions
- Increased competitiveness

Tools used in TQM

Tool	Purpose
Cause and effect diagram/Fishbone diagram	Identify and analyze causes of a problem
Checklists	Gathering of data
Flowcharts	Document detailed steps of a process
Scatter diagrams	Relation between two variables
Control charts	Identify variations in process
Histograms	Graphical display of frequency distribution of data
Pareto analysis	Degree of importance of each element

2.5 TQM IN DRUG INDUSTRY

Pharmaceutical literature does not offer any common definition for the term 'quality'. The idea implied in most definitions is the idea that the drug product has to meet customer needs. Customers cannot really assess the quality of their drugs and this is the reason why governments have to step in with rules and regulations to ensure the quality of medicines.

A study of the history of drug regulations reveals that most laws were enacted in response to tragedies that occurred when patients received drugs that were contaminated or not properly processed or incorrectly labeled. This led to a focus by drug makers on Quality Control – the process of testing the quality of products manufactured in their facilities.

As time evolved, and pharmaceutical processes grew more complex, it gradually came to be realized that no process is perfect all the time, and there are drifts from the normal functioning. The best of testing methods may miss detecting a problem because the destructive nature of the testing means only few samples drawn at random can be tested. Thus, there was a realization that relying on mere testing of products at the end of the manufacturing process is an ineffective (and costly) way of trying to ensure quality.

According to regulatory bodies across the world, high quality drug products are those that can be relied upon to deliver the desired clinical effects with consistency. Consumers of medicines need to know for sure that the drug product they are consuming are of good quality, safe for consumption, and will be effective in relieving them of their ailment. This quality can be guaranteed only if the products have it built into them right from the very first stage of design of the product and process. Realization of this basic principle led to the International Conference on Harmonization (ICH) in 2002, introducing a hitherto unheard of term in the drug processing field – the concept of 'Quality by Design' or QbD.

2.5.1 Quality by Design

The ICH guideline Q8 (R2) Pharmaceutical Development defines QbD as, "A systematic approach to development that begins with predefined objectives, emphasizes product, process understanding and process control, based on sound science and quality risk management."

To achieve the objective of QbD, it is important to understand product characteristics and study process characteristics using a combination of prior knowledge and experimental studies. From this data generated during product development, it becomes possible to decide which quality parameters in starting materials are the most important, and which critical processing factors need to be controlled to achieve a product with all the desired quality attributes.

The ICH Q10 guideline says that a Pharmaceutical Quality System is one that "assures that the desired product quality is routinely met, suitable process performance is achieved, the set of controls are appropriate, improvement opportunities are identified and evaluated, and the body of knowledge is continually expanded."

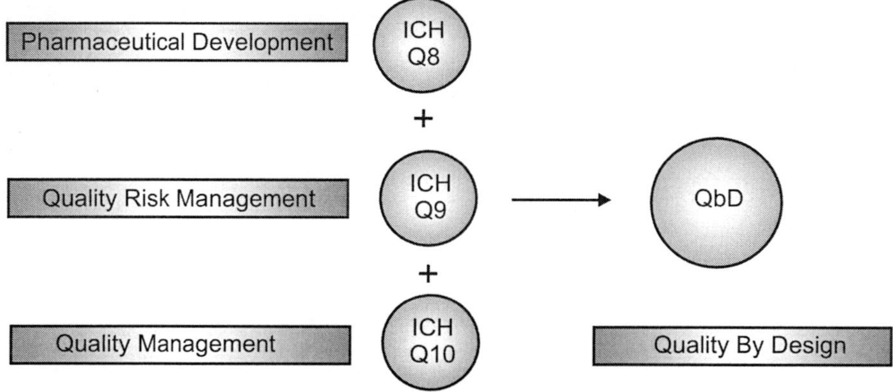

Fig. 2.1: Quality by Design

In other words, a robust pharmaceutical quality system is the key to supplying customers with high quality drugs. Such a system has the following characteristics:

- Aligned with requirements of current Good Manufacturing Practices (cGMP)
- Science-based and risk-based
- Comprehensive
- Proactive and accountable

Developing such pharmaceutical quality systems is the key to meeting patient requirements in an efficient manner. Because they deliver consistent quality, these systems also serve to increase the confidence of regulatory bodies about the organization's commitment to quality.

REVIEW QUESTIONS

1. Name the key thinkers of the quality movement and write about their concepts of quality.
2. Define TQM and discuss its advantages.
3. List the key elements of TQM and the tools it uses.
4. Explain how TQM principles are applied in the pharmaceutical industry.
5. Write a brief note about the concept of Quality by Design (QbD) in pharma industry.

☞ ☞ ☞

Chapter ...3

INTERNATIONAL CONFERENCE ON HARMONIZATION (ICH)

Objectives:

Upon completion of this section, the student should be able to

- Define the term 'ICH' and its purpose.
- Explain how the concept of harmonization was adopted in practice.
- Describe the organizational setup of ICH.
- List and explain the steps in the harmonization process.
- Explain the important ICH guidelines.
- List the ICH Quality guideline components.
- Outline stability testing guidelines as per ICH.

Introduction

In the 1980s, the pharmaceutical industry had begun expanding beyond domestic markets of individual countries, thanks to globalization. Legislations regarding quality standards of drugs were becoming more complex the world over, and it was becoming difficult for a manufacturer located in one country to match the specific drug regulatory requirements of another country to which they wished to export medicines. Regulators of one country were focused on their regulations and any products that didn't meet their requirements were rejected. Considering the increasingly international nature of the pharmaceutical market, drug regulators decided to work in collaboration, and this led to the birth of the International Conference on Harmonization (ICH).

3.1 ICH AND ITS PURPOSE

The full form of ICH is "International Conference on Harmonization of Technical Requirements for Registration of Pharmaceuticals for Human Use." This body was set up to bring together representatives of pharmaceutical industry and regulatory bodies to discuss technical and scientific aspects of registration of drugs. As the pharmaceutical industry grew more international, the differences in technical requirements across countries meant that drug makers had to spend lot of time and money to duplicate test procedures if they wanted to market their products at an international level. It started becoming important to make safe and effective drugs available to patients all over the world without the delays caused by regulations not matching across regulatory bodies of the different countries. Thus, a need was felt to rationalize and harmonize drug regulations, and this resulted in the inception of ICH in 1990.

Purpose of ICH may be summarized as follows:

- Ensuring quality, safety and efficacy of drugs.
- Harmonization of drug technical requirements.
- Avoid duplication of human clinical trials.
- Reduce use of animal testing but without a compromise on evaluating efficacy and safety of drugs.

3.2 HISTORY OF ICH

The European Commission pioneered the harmonization concept of pharmaceuticals in the 1980s as it moved towards developing a single market. Observing the success of this, discussions began between the United States, Europe and Japan to explore the possibility of harmonization.

During the World Health Organization's Conference of Drug Regulatory Authorities in 1989 in Paris, an action plan was drawn up for this harmonization. Drug authorities then reached out to the International Federation of Pharmaceutical Manufacturers and Associations (IFPMA) to decide about an international, joint industry-regulatory body initiative.

In April 1990, a meeting was held at Brussels, resulting in the birth of ICH. Representatives of industry associations and regulatory agencies of Europe, US and Japan met to plan an International Conference.

During the first Steering Committee meeting of ICH, the stakeholders reached an agreement about the terms of reference. They decided that the three criteria on which approval and authorization for new medicines would be given would be Quality, Safety and Efficacy. It was agreed that harmonization would focus on topics falling under these three critical criteria.

Over the years after its inception, ICH has evolved and grown to make greater harmonization possible to ensure development of effective, safe, high quality medicines and their easy registration.

The ICH also developed the concept of Common Technical Document (CTD) and Medical Dictionary for Regulatory Activities (MedDRA).

One of the biggest successes of ICH was the introduction of the concept of Quality by Design (QbD) to the pharmaceutical industry in 2009.

Organizational changes were made in October 2015 and now, ICH comprises 16 Members and 32 Observers.

Founding Members of ICH:

Member countries: United States, Japan and European Union

Regulatory Representatives:

1. European Commission (EC) and European Medicines Agency (EMA).
2. United States Food and Drug Administration (USFDA).
3. Japan's Ministry of Health, Labour and Welfare (MHLW).

Industrial Representatives:

1. EU's European Federation of Pharmaceutical Industries and Associations (EFPIA).
2. USA's Pharmaceutical Research and Manufacturers of America (PhRMA).
3. Japan's Pharmaceutical Manufacturers Association (JPMA).

3.3 PROCESS OF HARMONIZATION

The harmonization activities of ICH may fall into one of four categories : Formal ICH Procedure, Q & A Procedure, Revision Procedure and Maintenance Procedure.

ICH Procedures

Type of Procedure	Deals with
Formal ICH Procedure	New topic for harmonization
Q & A Procedure	Clarification for an existing ICH Guideline
Revision Procedure	Adding new information to an existing ICH Guideline
Maintenance Procedure	Changes to be made to maintain a guideline

First, a Concept Paper is prepared for the activity to be harmonized. This is a brief summary of the concept being proposed. Sometimes, a business plan may also be prepared to highlight the cost : benefit ratio of the harmonizing activity.

The formal ICH procedure then begins, in the following steps:

Step 1: Building consensus:

Based on the objectives specified in the Concept Paper, a working group prepares a consensus draft called the Technical Document. The working group's technical experts sign off on this, and the Step 1 Experts Technical Document is submitted to the ICH Assembly with a request for adoption.

Step 2: (a) Based on the report:

Assembly confirms that the scientific consensus exists for the technical issues, and the Technical Document may proceed further for regulatory consultation.

(b) This draft guideline is examined and endorsed by regulatory members of the ICH Assembly.

Step 3: This happens in three different stages:

Consultation, discussion and finalization of the Expert Draft Guideline by regulatory members at different levels.

Stage 1: The draft guideline goes to the different ICH regions for discussion in their respective regulatory regions.

Stage 2: All comments obtained during stage 1 are addressed by the expert working group and after discussion, consensus is reached to prepare the step 3 Experts Draft Guideline.

Stage 3: This draft guideline is finalized and signed by the ICH regulatory member experts. The document is sent to ICH Assembly regulatory members for further proceeding to step 4.

Step 4: ICH Assembly regulatory members agree that sufficient scientific consensus exists on the draft guideline, and it gets adopted as the ICH Harmonized Guideline.

Step 5: ICH Harmonized Guideline is implemented in all the ICH regions through their respective regulatory procedures. Information about when it has become effective is sent to the ICH Assembly and published on the ICH website.

3.4 ICH GUIDELINES: QUALITY, SAFETY, EFFICACY, MULTIDISCIPLINARY (QSEM)

The ICH guidelines are covered under four headings under the acronym QSEM – Quality, Safety, Efficacy and Multidisciplinary.

(a) Quality guidelines: These guidelines cover the areas of quality of drug products such as impurity testing and stability studies and a flexible approach to quality on the basis of GMP risk management.

(b) Safety guidelines: They help to detect potential risks such as genotoxicity, carcinogenicity and reprotoxicity. For example, the ICH came up with a non-clinical test methodology to evaluate QT interval prolongation which is probably the most significant reason why drugs have been withdrawn in recent times.

(c) Efficacy guidelines: These guidelines provide guidance about designing, conducting, safety aspects and reporting of clinical trials for pharmaceutical products. Novel drug products derived from biotechnology and genomic/pharmacogenetic techniques for targeted drug delivery are also covered.

(d) Multidisciplinary guidelines: Topics in the pharmaceutical field that do not fit into any of the above categories are covered under this area. This guideline also includes details of (MedDRA), CTD and standards such as Electronic Standards for the Transfer of Regulatory Information (ESTRI)

3.5 QUALITY GUIDELINES

Out of all these guidelines, the one most relevant to us is the Quality guidelines. The areas covered under this are labeled from Q1 to Q11 and deal with different aspects of Quality Assurance (QA) relating to pharmaceuticals. Stability testing, analytical validation, impurities, quality systems, risk management and GMP are some of the most important areas covered.

Guideline	Subpart	Area covered
Q1 Stability	Q1 A	Stability testing of new drug substances and products.
	Q1 B	Photostability testing of new drug substances and products.
	Q1 C	Stability testing for new dosage forms.
	Q1 D	Bracketing and matrixing designs for stability testing of new drug substances and products.
	Q1 E	Evaluation of stability data.
	Q1 F	Stability data package for registration applications in climatic zones III and IV.
Q2		Validation of analytical procedures.
Q3 Impurities	Q3 A	Impurities in new drug substances.
	Q3 B	Impurities in new drug products.
	Q3 C	Guidelines for residual solvents.
	Q3 D	Guidelines for elemental impurities.
Q4 Pharmacopoeias	Q4 A	Pharmacopoeial harmonization.
	Q4 B	Evaluation and recommendation of pharmacopoeial texts for use in ICH regions.
Q5 Quality of biotechnological products	Q5 A	Viral safety evaluation of biotechnology products derived from cell lines of human or animal origin.
	Q5 B	Analysis of expression construct in cells used for production of r-DNA derived protein products.
	Q5 C	Stability testing of biotechnological/biological products.
	Q5 D	Derivation and characterization of cell substrates used for production of biotechnological/biological products.
	Q5 E	Comparability of biotechnological / biological products subject to changes in their manufacturing process.

... (Contd.)

Guideline	Subpart	Area covered
Q6 Specifications	Q6 A	Test procedures and acceptance criteria for new drug substances and new drug products: Chemical substances.
	Q6 B	Test procedures and acceptance criteria for biotechnological/ biological products.
Q7		Good manufacturing practices for Active pharmaceutical ingredients.
Q8		Pharmaceutical development.
Q9		Quality risk management.
Q10		Pharmaceutical quality system.
Q11		Development and manufacture of drug substances (chemical and biological entities).

3.6 ICH GUIDELINES FOR STABILITY

The ICH guidelines for stability testing define what information must be provided at the time of applying to register a new drug molecule. These guidelines were first adopted in 1993. After revision and updation, the current version in use called Q1A(R2) has been adopted since 2003. This guideline harmonizes the drug registration process for all drugs in the USA, Japan and the EU. This means a drug registered in one of these regions will not require repeated stability testing when to be sold in any of the other two regions.

Stability testing is important because drug products must be stable when administered to the patients. If an unstable product degrades into toxic metabolites, or if activity of the drug reduces below 85% of the label claim, there can be serious therapy failures that may even result in death. Stability testing also provides data to choose the formulation parameters, excipients and the right container-closure system to ensure safe and effective quality products that retain activity throughout shelf life.

The stability testing data must provide information about how the drug molecule changes over time under different storage conditions. This gives insight into how light, heat and humidity will influence the chemical nature of the product. Drugs which are unstable will need specific storage conditions if they have to remain effective. Therefore, it is vital to perform stress testing to study and document the conditions that lead to degradation of the drug molecule. This information is used to arrive at the shelf life of the drug and what conditions will be optimal for storage of the product.

3.6.1 Types of Stability Testing

1. **Real-time testing:** This involves testing drug product for a longer duration to find out what is the maximum product degradation when stored as recommended.
2. **Accelerated stability testing:** Here, product is subjected to stress in the form of higher temperatures, moisture, agitation, light, pH, and packaging conditions to study its degradation profile.
3. **Retained sample stability testing:** This is testing of samples retained from each batch that has been sent into the market.
4. **Cyclic temperature stress testing:** Not routinely used. It involves subjecting the products to temperature stresses in a way to mimic likely market storage conditions.

3.6.2 Stability Testing Protocol

This is the written document that describes all major requirements of a well-controlled stability study for a given drug substance or drug product. The basic information to be included in a stability test protocol includes:

- Batch selection – how many batches to be tested
- Containers and closures that must be used for the testing
- Different positions in which product containers must be kept during testing
- Frequency of drawing samples for analysis
- Overall sampling plan – when and how much to sample and from where
- Test storage conditions based on climatic zone where drug will be used
- Parameters to be tested to evaluate product stability – mainly the ones expected to change after storage
- Methods to be used for testing, and their validation
- Acceptance criteria for result values, and for degradation products

The data obtained by performing the stability studies is used for expiration dating of the drug product and to determine its shelf life.

3.6.3 Overview of ICH Stability Guidelines Contents

Some of the areas covered by the ICH guidelines on stability testing include:

- **Stress testing:** Study of degradation pathways, effects of change in temperature, relative humidity, pH changes, susceptibility to be degraded by moisture (hydrolysis).
- **Photostability testing:** Study of effect of light on drug chemistry.
- **Batch selection for stability testing:** Not less than 3 primary batches of drug substance.
- **Testing of container closure system:** At least thrice; once in 3 months in first year, once in 6 months during the second year and then annually.
- Storage conditions for the drug substance and product.
- Storage instructions with respect to different regions and climatic zones, and labeling requirements regarding storage region-wise.

Thanks to the harmonization process of ICH, there are now more than 50 harmonized guidelines. This had led to streamlining of the research and development process and in turn, made it easier to develop and market new medicines to patients all over the globe. There are certainly concerns that non-ICH members are not consulted in the decision-making; however, the educational material provided by ICH is largely beneficial for such countries to streamline their own R&D and drug manufacturing efforts.

The membership of ICH has grown over the years of its inception. For ICH to continue to grow and stay relevant, it is necessary to have greater participation from more countries across the world. Future plans must consider the involvement of non-ICH members, recognizing and finding ways to overcome the challenges that developing nations face in using the ICH guidelines.

REVIEW QUESTIONS

1. Define ICH and discuss how it came into being.
2. Explain the process of harmonization adopted for preparing new ICH guidelines.
3. Discuss the QSEM guidelines as per ICH.
4. Describe the ICH Quality guidelines.
5. Write a note on the ICH guidelines for stability testing of pharmaceutical products.

Chapter ...4

PHARMACEUTICAL QUALITY BY DESIGN

Objectives:

Upon completion of this section, the student should be able to

- Define the concept of Quality by Design (QbD).
- Connect the concept of QbD to the ICH guidelines from which it evolved.
- Describe the elements of QbD.
- Explain process flow and design in QbD.
- List control strategies used in QbD.
- Explain important tools used in QbD.
- List the advantages and challenges of using QbD.

Introduction

Pharmaceutical manufacturers take several steps to make sure they produce good quality products. Yet, it has been found that several concerns plague the drug development and manufacturing processes.

The pioneer in quality, Dr. Joseph M. Juran was the first to develop the concept of Quality by Design (QbD). He proposed that quality must be designed into the product; if this is done, there will not be any of the quality crises that one commonly encounters.

In a report titled, 'Pharmaceutical Quality for the 21st Century: A Risk-Based Approach,' the US Food and Drug Administration (FDA) furthered these ideas, and provided an initiative to address quality issues. Through collaboration with major pharma companies, the FDA created a set of guidance documents on the concept of Quality by Design (QbD). These were then accepted by the International Conference on Harmonization (ICH) to streamline and regulate the process of drug development and regulatory filing related to drug manufacture.

The main idea behind the QbD concept is that a process must be designed to produce quality products. This becomes possible only when the process and product are both thoroughly understood, and the risks involved in its manufacturing are studied carefully, and steps are outlined to mitigate such risks. This QbD approach is significantly different from the traditional, empirical approach that emphasised on testing of quality in the end products.

4.1 DEFINITION

The ICH guideline Q8 (R2) Pharmaceutical Development defines the term Quality by Design (QbD) as "a systematic approach to development that begins with predefined objectives, emphasizes product, process understanding and process control, based on sound science and quality risk management."

4.2 OVERVIEW

From the above definition, it is clear that pharmaceutical QbD is an organized approach to drug development. It starts with pre-determined objectives with an emphasis on understanding the process and product. It focuses on controlling the process and product on the basis of sound science and the concept of quality risk management.

Some of the key objectives of QbD include:

- Achieving meaningful quality specifications for the product on the basis of clinical performance.
- Enhancing process capability, and reducing product defects and variability by improving the process and product design and control.
- To promote root cause analysis and manage any changes of drug product after it has been approved.
- To improve efficiency of the processes involved in product development and manufacturing.

Thus, in the pharmaceutical QbD approach, first, critical quality characteristics (from the patient's point of view) need to be identified. These characteristics are then translated into critical quality attributes (CQAs) of the drug product. Next, a relationship is established between manufacturing process variables and CQAs. Successful control of these variables ensures the consistent delivery of a quality drug product with all desired CQAs to the patient.

ICH documents on which QbD is based

ICH document	Subject	Details
ICH Q8 (R2)	Pharmaceutical Development.	Drug product development using science principles.
ICH Q9	Quality Risk Management.	How to assess, control, review and manage quality risks.
ICH Q10	Pharmaceutical Quality System.	Quality systems, how to improve process performance and product quality.
ICH Q11	Development and Manufacture of Drug Substances (Chemical Entities and Biotechnological/Biological Entities).	How to select starting materials, validate processes and control them.
ICH Q12	Technical and Regulatory Considerations for Pharmaceutical Product Lifecycle Management.	Regulatory factors in pharmaceutical products and life cycle change management.

4.3 ELEMENTS OF QbD

The elements of QbD include:

1. Quality Target Product Profile (QTPP) – it identifies the CQAs of drug product.
2. Product design and identifying Critical Material Attributes (CMAs).
3. Process design and identifying Critical Process Parameters (CPPs). This includes linking the CMAs and CPPs with CQAs.
4. Controls strategy : developing specifications for active pharmaceutical ingredients (APIs), excipients and final drug product; also controls for every step of the production process.
5. Process capabilities and continued improvement.

Flow of events in QbD

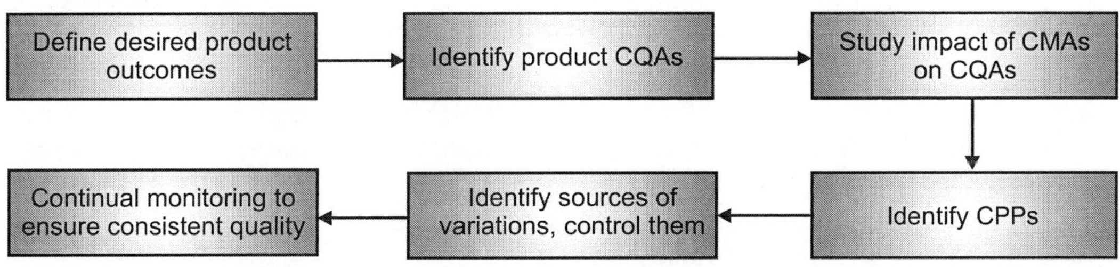

Fig. 4.1

Quality Target Product Profile (QTPP):

QTPP is a summary of the quality parameters that must be present in the drug product to ensure the desired quality is achieved. This is the basis on which product design will commence. When formulating the QTPP, the points to be considered include:

1. The intended use of the product, its route of administration, desired dosage form and system used for drug delivery.
2. Strength of the dose.
3. Container-closure system to be used.
4. Release of the therapeutic component and factors that will influence pharmacokinetic parameters (such as dissolution of drug) in the proposed dosage form.
5. Quality criteria for the final product – stability, purity, sterility, drug release etc.

Critical Quality Attributes (CQAs):

After finalizing the QTPP, it is possible to identify the CQAs of the drug product. CQAs are properties of the finished product – physical, chemical, biological or microbiological – that must lie within certain range, limits or distribution, in order to ensure that desired quality of product is attained.

Some examples of quality attributes of drug products include identity of drug, assay values, content uniformity, drug release profile, degradation products, microbial levels, moisture content and physical properties such as size, colour, shape and friability. Not all of them may be critical attributes. Whether an attribute is critical or not depends upon the severity of the damage that will be caused if the product falls outside the acceptable range for that particular attribute.

Product Design:

A well designed product is one that meets patients' requirements and this can be confirmed through clinical studies. Such a product will maintain its performance throughout its shelf life, and this can be confirmed by stability studies. Thus, product design must be geared towards developing a robust product that delivers the desired QTPP over the entire shelf life of the product.

For good product design, it is important to study the following in detail:
- Physical, chemical and biological characteristics of the drug (examples: particle size, polymorphism, solubility, melting point, pKa, oxidative stability, partition coefficient, bioavailability, membrane permeability etc.).
- Type of excipients and their grade, and details of intrinsic excipient variability (common excipients such as binders, diluents, disintegrants, glidants, colouring agents, sweeteners, suspending agents, film coatings, preservatives, flavours etc.).
- Interactions of drug substances with excipients by carrying out drug-excipient compatibility testing.
- The critical material attributes (CMAs) of both drug and excipients to ensure development of a robust formulation.

CMA vs CQA

CMA: Physical, chemical, biological or microbiological characteristic of **raw material** that must lie within appropriate limits or range to ensure desired quality.

CQA: Physical, chemical, biological or microbiological characteristic of **drug product intermediates or finished drug products** that must lie within appropriate limits or range to ensure desired quality.

Process Design:

Manufacturing process for a drug product is made up of a set of unit operations run in a particular sequence, to give the final product. The term unit operation refers to any activity where there is a physical or chemical change in the substance. Milling, mixing, granulation, drying, tablet compression, coating, are all examples of unit operations in tablet manufacture.

Processes must be designed in such a way that each unit operation is performed as expected to deliver the necessary product. For this, it is important to:

(a) Identify the critical causes of variations.

(b) Manage these variations during the process.

(c) Predict quality attributes of the product with accuracy and reliability.

Any parameter whose variability can have an adverse impact on a CQA, is critical to the process, and called as Critical Process Parameter (CPP). All CPPs for a given process must be first identified; then they must be monitored and regulated to make sure that desired quality products are produced.

Process robustness studies must be performed to check if the process can tolerate variability in the input materials and processing parameters and still deliver a product of acceptable quality. These studies will also serve to identify CPPs which have an impact on drug quality.

Evaluation of CMAs, CPPs and CQAs for unit operation of tablet compression

CMAs	CPPs	CQAs
Particle size distribution	Type of press	Appearance of tablet
Proportion of oversize/fines	Design of hopper, vibration, height	Tablet weight and uniformity
Shape of granules		Hardness
Cohesive properties	Feed mechanism 0-force feed/gravity feed, rotational direction	Friability
Hardness		Content uniformity
Density values – bulk/tapped/true	Tool design – metal quality, score configuration	Thickness
Electrostatic properties		Tablet density/porosity
Brittleness	Maximum punch load	Defects
Moisture content	Pressing speed	Disintegration time
Polymorphism	Compression force (pre, main)	Moisture content
	Penetration depth of punch	Dissolution profile
	Dwell time	
	Ejection force	

How to understand processes?

1. List all process parameters that may impact the process performance
2. Using scientific knowledge and risk assessment, identify the parameters that are potentially high risk
3. Establish ranges for these high-risk potential parameters
4. Design and carry out experiments to test these parameters
5. Obtain experimental data and analyze it using first principle models to confirm how critical the process parameter is. Connect CPPs and CMAs to CQAs wherever possible
6. Develop a control mechanism by defining acceptable ranges for critical parameters and non-critical parameters.

Control Strategy:

The data generated during developmental studies must be used to set up a control strategy. It is common to have controls at three levels as follows:

Level 1: Automated engineering controls are used for real-time monitoring of CQAs of the output materials. The system is designed to monitor the input material attributes, and adjust the process parameters automatically, so that CQAs consistently meet the predetermined acceptance criteria. Process Analytical Technology (PAT) systems are an example of this type of control.

Level 2: Here, the emphasis is on understanding the process and product, and designing it with control over the pharmaceutical process. This is QbD and it allows the control of variables, and thus, ensures drug product quality.

Level 3: This strategy depends on detailed testing of end-product as seen in conventional pharmaceutical manufacturing. As the sources of variability have not been identified, and there is no study of CMAs and CPPs on the quality of drug product, the likelihood of product problems is high.

In real life situations, it is best to combine level 1 and level 2 control strategies to arrive at a hybrid approach that involves:

1. Controlling attributes of input material based on a study of their impact on product quality and the processability.
2. Establishing product specifications.
3. Controlling unit operations that have biggest impact on product quality.
4. Testing in-process, in real time instead of relying on end-product testing.
5. Setting up a monitoring program to verify control over the process and product.

Process Capability and Continued Improvement:

Process capability is a measure of the level of inherent variability shown by a stable process that is under control, when compared with the established acceptance criteria. Variability may be short-term or long-term, and the QbD program must result in identification and reduction of the variations that impact the quality of product.

Continuous improvement methods need to be adopted to remove these sources of variability. This includes several activities in different phases such as:

1. Defining the problem and setting up specific goals
2. Measuring key areas of the process and collecting necessary data
3. Data analysis to find cause-effect relationships
4. Use results of data analysis to optimize the process
5. Perform pilot runs to check optimized process capabilities
6. Monitor processes to make sure they stay in a state of statistical control

4.4 QUALITY BY DESIGN TOOLS

Quality by Design relies on the use of certain tools. These include prior knowledge, risk assessment, mechanistic models, design of experiments and data analysis, and process analytical technology.

4.4.1 Prior Knowledge

As per ICH guidelines, prior knowledge is the information or knowledge or skills that have been acquired through previous experience of similar processes and published information. This tool can be used at the beginning of the developmental process and may be regularly updated using data generated during the process. Prior knowledge can be applied as a part of control strategies, in relation to QTPP and CQAs. However, it is important to avoid too much reliance on prior knowledge as it may result in a loss of control over the manufacturing process. It is best to use this tool to confirm data rather than to build data from scratch.

4.4.2 Risk Assessment

As per ICH Q9, quality risk management must be done before development studies to detect the high-risk variables that have an impact on drug product quality. Risk evaluation must be done on the basis of scientific knowledge and is often used to determine critical variables. These variables must then be further investigated through experimentation, so that a control strategy may be established.

Some of the common risk assessment tools used are flowcharts, fault tree analysis, failure mode effects analysis, hazard analysis and critical control points, risk ranking and filtering etc.

FMEA and HACCP

Failure Mode Effect Analysis (FMEA):

Failure mode refers to the defects or errors in a material, equipment, design or process. After establishing these failure modes, the tool evaluates their effects, and ranks them in order of priority. This method may also include a study of how critical the consequences of the failures are. Sometimes, Ishikawa diagrams (fishbone/cause-and-effect) are also used.

Hazard Analysis and Critical Control Points (HACCP):

Hazards that can cause safety and quality issues are identified (for example, hygiene of personnel, material flow, environmental aspects, process design, manufacturing steps). Preventive measures for each of these are established. Next, critical control points are determined for these hazards, and limits are established. A system is set up to monitor these critical control points, and corrective actions to be taken when these are not in a state of control, are determined. Finally, record-keeping systems are set up to monitor and confirm that the HACCP system itself is working as expected.

4.4.3 Design of Experiments

This tool involves setting up a series of structured tests where changes to the variables of a process are made in a planned manner. Then, the impact of these changes on a chosen output is assessed. This tool is very effective in identifying all the factors that together impact the output responses. The interaction of the variable factors can also be quantified.

4.4.4 Process Analytical Technology (PAT)

The US FDA defines PAT as "A system for designing, analyzing, and controlling manufacturing through timely measurements (i.e., during processing) of critical quality and performance attributes of raw and in-process materials and processes, with the goal of ensuring final product quality.

PAT allows real-time monitoring of CMAs, CPPs or CQAs to demonstrate that the process is in a state of control. It enables online measurements that are very useful to detect failures, and also allows adjustment of the operational parameters when variations that have a negative impact on product quality are detected.

PAT includes a wide variety of tools to acquire physical, chemical, microbiological, analytical and mathematical data and risk analysis. By creating an interface of process with instrument, and also a feedback loop that can modify processing conditions, PAT helps to control process parameters as well as product quality.

Advantages of QbD:

1. Better assurance of product quality due to improved process design and better quality risk management during the manufacturing process.
2. Innovation and increased efficiency and reduced potential for errors lead to cost savings.
3. Improves regulatory compliance and streamlines change management.
4. Real time testing during the process ensures faster releases as compared to traditional end-testing of finished products.

Challenges to QbD:

1. Requires cultural change in the organizational approach to quality.
2. Expensive, requires management support.
3. Calls for collaboration between departments and there may be resource/workload limitations.

In conclusion, we can understand QbD as a quality system that helps to manage the life cycle of a product. It aims at designing a capable process through better product and process understanding and through this, hopes to reduce the risk of patients taking drug products. The emphasis in QbD is on continuous improvement, building on past experience, using risk management approaches, and documenting knowledge to achieve high quality drug products that consistently meet their quality specifications.

REVIEW QUESTIONS

1. Define the term 'Quality by Design'. List its advantages and demerits.
2. Explain how the concept of QbD is related to the ICH guidelines.
3. List and explain a few important QbD tools used in the pharma industry.
4. Define the terms QTPP, CQA, CMA and CPP in Quality by Design.
5. Write a note on FMEA and HACCP.
6. Discuss the concept of PAT and its advantages.

✍ ✍ ✍

Chapter ...5

INTRODUCTION TO ISO 9000 AND ISO 14000

Objectives:

Upon completion of this section, the student should be able to

- Outline the development of ISO standards.
- Explain the aims and principles of ISO.
- Describe ISO 9000 and ISO 14000 families.
- List the elements of ISO 9000 certification.
- Explain the benefits of ISO certification.

Introduction

Quality is a very important requirement for any product because it is one of the biggest factors determining how successful it will be in achieving customer satisfaction. Quality is often described as the extent to which a product or service meets the existing standards or requirements. Quality has become the catchword across industries and professions and quality management systems are being developed by the day to ensure better business processes. One such quality management system is provided by the International Organization for Standardization which is abbreviated as ISO.

5.1 HISTORY OF ISO

Every country has its own standards for every industry. But in an increasingly globalized business scenario, a need was felt for a common set of standards to make it easier for businesses to sell their products anywhere in the world. Against this background, about 65 delegates from 25 countries met in London in 1946 at the Institute of Civil Engineers. The agenda was to facilitate the unification of industrial standards at an international level. The following year, in February 1947, the non-governmental organization called International Organization for Standardization (ISO) was born, and 67 technical committees were set up.

5.2 OVERVIEW OF ISO

From the 25 members who met to initiate this process, ISO has grown to a huge network of more than 160 member countries who represent their nation's standards organizations. The ISO headquarters is located in Geneva, Switzerland. The ISO is considered the world's largest organization involved with developing voluntary international standards. In this role, the ISO helps to facilitate global trade by creating common standards across countries. Over the years since it began functioning, ISO has set more than 20,000 standards in different areas right from manufacturing and agriculture to food safety and healthcare.

5.3 AIM OF ISO INTERNATIONAL STANDARDS

The purpose of the International Standards developed by ISO is to ensure that products and services are safe, reliable and of good quality. For business, they are strategic tools that reduce costs by minimizing waste and errors and increasing productivity. They help companies to access new markets, level the playing field for developing countries and facilitate free and fair global trade.

Organizations often wish to certify their quality systems but the ISO does not issue any such certificates. However, there are registered institutions and accreditation bodies who are qualified to perform the certification on behalf of ISO. An organization that meets the requirements of certification is issued an ISO certificate for the standards to which it conforms, and the certificate is valid for 3 years.

Principles on which ISO standards are based

- Customer-focus
- Leadership
- Engagement of people
- Process approach
- Continual improvement
- Evidence-based decision making
- Relationship management

5.4 ISO 9000 FAMILY

The ISO 9000 family is probably the best known of ISO standards. It is the set of International Standards that lays down the framework for a quality management system. The purpose of these is to guide organizations with the tools required to make sure that their services or products meet quality requirements and drive the process of continued quality improvement. These standards are universal and may be applied to organizations in any industry and of any size.

ISO 9000 standards were published first in 1987. Major revisions were made in 2000 and later in 2008. The most recent versions are the ones published in 2015.

Some of the important standards in this family include :

ISO 9000:2015 – basic concepts and vocabulary (definitions)

ISO 9001: 2015 – requirements of a quality management system

ISO 9004: 2018 – continuous improvement of quality management systems

ISO 19011: 2011 – guidelines for internal and external audits of quality management systems.

While ISO 9000 is the standard that describes the quality management system, it is ISO 9001 standard that describes what requirements must be met to achieve that system in the organization. Thus, certification is given under ISO 9001 and not ISO 9000.

5.4.1 Criteria to get ISO 9001 Certification

- Organization must follow the guidelines laid down in the ISO 9001 standard.
- It must meet its own requirements.
- It must meet regulatory and statutory requirements.
- It must meet customer requirements.
- It must document its performance.

5.4.2 Benefits of ISO 9001 Certification

There are several advantages of ISO 9000 certification and these impact all aspects of an organization. The most important ones include:

1. Increased credibility from the ISO certification which increases the organization's marketability.
2. The rigorous certification process exposes deficiencies in the organization and when these are addressed, it leads to significant cost savings in terms of time and money.
3. The certification helps to improve quality of products and processes resulting in better/higher customer satisfaction.
4. Management control improves because of all the documentation and self-assessment involved in the registration process.
5. Communication and interactions between the different departments in the organization improve creating better team spirit.
6. As organizations move to improve their quality, the risk of product-liability begins to reduce.

Important elements of ISO 9000

1. Management responsibility
2. Quality system
3. Contract review
4. Design control
5. Document and data control
6. Purchasing
7. Control of customer-supplied product
8. Product identification and traceability
9. Process control

10. Inspection and testing
11. Control of inspection, measuring and test equipment
12. Inspection and test status
13. Control of non-conforming material
14. Corrective and preventive action
15. Handling, storage, packaging, preservation and delivery
16. Control of quality records
17. Internal quality audits
18. Training
19. Servicing
20. Statistical techniques

5.5 ISO 14000

ISO 14000 family comprises the international standards, technical reports and guides for environmental management by organizations. They specify the requirements necessary to set up an environmental management policy, plan and implement environmental objectives, determine the impact of products or services on the environment and conducting corrective actions and management review. By working towards ISO 14000 certification, organizations can reduce the negative impact of their processes on the environment (air, land or water).

Some of the important standards in this family include:

ISO 14004: 2016 – Environmental management systems – general guidelines on implementation.

ISO 14006: 2011 – Environmental management systems – guidelines to incorporate ecodesign.

ISO 14031: 2013 – Environmental Management – environmental performance evaluation guidelines.

ISO 14064: 2006 – Greenhouse gases standards.

ISO 14020: 2000 – Environmental Labels and Declarations – general principles.

5.5.1 Aim of ISO 14000 Standards

The ISO 14000 standards were developed as industries recognized the need for standardization in the area of environmental management. They aim at ensuring organizations promote environmental management systems that are effective.

The first standard for environmental management system was the BS 7750 that was published in 1992. In 1996, ISO published the ISO 14000 family of standards, which was subsequently revised in 2004 and the latest version available is of 2015. ISO 14001 is the standard to which organizations can get certified.

5.5.2 Benefits of ISO 14000

ISO 14000 certification has several benefits for organizations, such as:

1. It helps meet legal obligations towards environmental protection.
2. Resources are used more efficiently.
3. Waste is reduced.
4. Environmental impacts get measured.
5. Customer and stakeholder trust increases.
6. Environmental obligations are managed the right way.

ISO certifications are important for organizations because they provide customers with evidence of the company's commitment to quality. The standards have a process-oriented approach and look at how processes operate across departments and their interaction; they also help to focus on the most critical of products and services and therefore, are an effective check of the company's quality management systems.

REVIEW QUESTIONS

1. Define ISO and discuss its aims and principles.
2. Explain the history of ISO standards development.
3. What are the important elements of ISO 9000 certification?
4. Discuss the benefits of ISO certification for a pharmaceutical company.
5. Explain the ISO 9000 family of standards.
6. What is the significance of the ISO 14000 family of standards?

✍ ✍ ✍

Chapter ...6

NABL ACCREDITATION

Objectives:

Upon completion of this section, the student should be able to

- Define the meaning of accreditation.
- Explain advantages of accreditation over ISO certification.
- Describe Indian regulations regarding accreditation for laboratories.
- List and explain the steps in the accreditation process for Conformity Assessment Bodies (CABs).
- Describe the preparation process required before applying for accreditation.

6.1 INTRODUCTION

Laboratory studies form an important part of assessing the quality of products. For test results to be accepted at national and international levels, they must be proven to be reliable. This is possible only when the systems in those laboratories meet certain quality requirements. The process of certifying this is called as accreditation.

Definition:

Accreditation of laboratories is a process through which an authorized, independent agency examines and certifies the competence and quality systems of a laboratory based on particular predefined standards.

Accreditation provides formal recognition of the technical competence of a laboratory for particular measurements or tests based on results from a third party assessment.

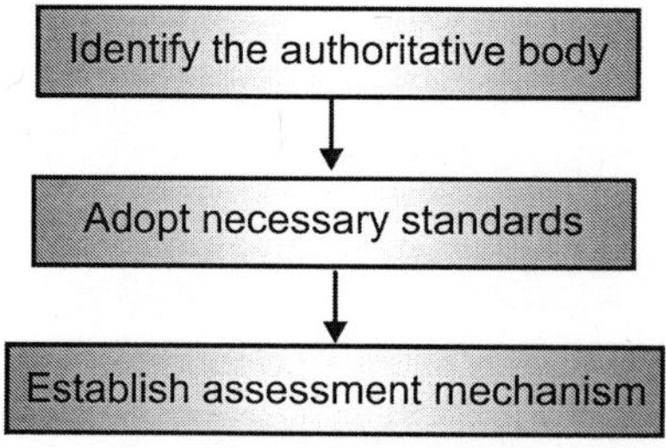

Fig. 6.1: Accreditation Process

Advantages of Accreditation:

1. Higher level of confidence in calibration/testing reports that the laboratory issues.
2. Increased business with greater customer confidence in testing reports.

3. Improved control over laboratory operations to maintain a sound quality management system.

4. Guarantee of reliable test results, reducing the need for re-testing, resulting in savings.

5. Improved visibility in the market as a good quality service provider.

Accreditation versus ISO 9000 Certification:

Accreditation is recognition of the technical competence of a test service provider or Conformity Assessment Body (CAB). Thus, it is a step beyond system certification provided by ISO 9000. ISO certification will evaluate the CAB's system for quality management; however, it will not give any insight to its ability to provide accurate and reliable test data, or its technical competence in testing. By assessing the CAB for compliance with internationally accepted criteria, accreditation provides a greater level of information than mere ISO certification.

In most countries, accreditation for laboratories is mandatory; in India, however, it is a voluntary exercise.

India's Accreditation Body – NABL:

In India, the accreditation body is named the National Accreditation Board for Testing and Calibration Laboratories – NABL. This body is a signatory of the Mutual Recognition Agreement with the regional body called Asia Pacific Laboratory Accreditation Cooperation and the apex body called International Laboratory Accreditation Cooperation. By this, NABL accredited laboratories can also achieve international recognition.

NABL is an autonomous body that is under the Department of Science and Technology, Government of India. It was first established to provide accreditation to laboratories involved with testing and calibration. Later, its scope was extended to accreditation for clinical laboratories, too. This is the only accreditation body authorized by Government of India for the testing and calibration laboratories.

Standards:

Internationally, the acceptable standards for laboratories is ISO 15189. NABL provides accreditation in keeping with ISO/IEC 17025 : 2005 "General Requirements for the Competence of Testing and Calibration Laboratories" and ISO 15189 : 2012 'Medical laboratories — Requirements for quality and competence'.

Fields of CABs covered by NABL

Testing Laboratories	Calibration Laboratories	Medical Laboratories
Biological	Electro-Technical	Clinical Biochemistry
Chemical	Mechanical	Clinical Pathology
Electrical	Fluid Flow	Haematology & Immunohaematology

... (Contd.)

Testing Laboratories	Calibration Laboratories	Medical Laboratories
Electronics	Thermal & Optical	Microbiology & Serology
Fluid-Flow	Radiological	Histopathology
Mechanical		Cytopathology
Non-Destructive Testing		Genetics
Photometry		Nuclear Medicine (in-vitro tests only)
Radiological		
Thermal		
Forensic		
Proficiency Testing Providers		**Reference Material Producers**
Testing		Chemical Composition
Calibration		Biological & Clinical Properties
Medical		Physical Properties
Inspection		Engineering Properties
		Miscellaneous Properties

Source: NABL India website

How often accreditation must be done?

For it to be effective in maintaining quality performance and reliability of results, accreditation must be done periodically, at regular intervals. NABL accreditation has a validity period of 2 years. The CAB must apply for accreditation renewal a minimum of 6 months before the accreditation validity period expires.

Procedure for NABL Accreditation:

CABs must follow the following process to obtain accreditation:

Step 1: CAB applies in the prescribed form in triplicate and attach two copies of their quality manual describing their management system as per ISO or IEC guidelines as applicable. CAB also pays the application fee prescribed by NABL.

Step 2: On receiving application, quality manual and fee, NABL Secretariat issues an acknowledgement number with a unique ID number. This must be used for any correspondence. NABL scrutinizes the application and may ask for any clarification or information as necessary.

Step 3: NABL appoints a lead assessor who organizes a pre-assessment visit to the CAB premises. During this visit, any non-conformity in quality system implementation is evaluated.

This visit helps to evaluate:

(a) How prepared CAB is for the assessment?

(b) How many assessors will be required?

(c) Which key locations must be visited?

Step 4: Lead assessor submits a report of the pre-assessment visit to NABL Secretariat. A copy is sent to the CAB too.

Step 5: CAB takes corrective measures regarding the non-conformity pointed out in pre-assessment report. CAB sends a report on this to NABL Secretariat.

Step 6: Based on the satisfactoriness of the CAB's corrective actions, NABL sets up the assessment team after consulting with the CAB. Along with the lead assessor, this team will include experts in the fields in which accreditation is sought by the CAB. Sometimes, an observer may also be nominated.

Step 7: Assessment team visits the CABs site. It reviews their systems and verifies compliance with the relevant certification standards. The team evaluates the CABs technical competence, and identifies non-conformities that may be present.

Step 8: Assessment team prepares an assessment report, and based on the findings, recommends if accreditation may be granted or not. This report is sent to the NABL Secretariat. A copy of the report is given to the CAB at the end of the inspection.

Step 9: NABL examines the assessment report and initiates any follow-up action for non-conformities. It monitors the corrective actions taken by the CAB.

Step 10: Once all non-conformities have been addressed, the CAB is granted accreditation by the Chairman, NABL. The accreditation certificate will have the NABL hologram, unique number, discipline, and scope of accreditation along with the validity date.

If CAB does not agree with the decisions of the NABL, it may appeal to the Director, NABL with necessary information.

NABL will survey the accredited CAB annually to ensure they continue to comply with certification requirements.

Preparing for Accreditation:

When a CAB wishes to apply for accreditation, they must prepare in advance for the process. Here are some important steps to be performed.

1. Obtain NABL documents from the NABL Secretariat to get familiar with the assessment process and details required for the application.

2. Ensure training of one person by NABL on Quality Management System and Internal Audit.

3. Prepare a quality manual in keeping with the standards.

4. For each test/investigation done in the laboratory, prepare a Standard Operating Procedure (SOP).

5. Calibrate instruments and equipment used in testing; ensure correct environmental conditions are maintained in the laboratory.

6. Train personnel on documentation aspects.

7. Check the status of current technical competence and quality system by comparing with NABL standards and address deficiencies encountered.
8. Prepare Quality Manual and all other documents required by NABL.
9. Include Internal Quality Control (IQC) in sample analysis.
10. Take part in External Quality Assessment Schemes (EQAs).
11. Evaluate compliance with IQC and EQAs; take corrective actions where necessary.
12. Perform internal audit and management review to assess preparedness for NABL assessment.
13. After everything is satisfactory, apply for accreditation to NABL with the prescribed fees.

Laboratory testing is a vital component of the health care system. Accreditation is an efficient tool to assess the quality of laboratory services and is therefore highly beneficial to healthcare providers. For it to be effective in maintaining quality performance and reliability of results, accreditation must be done periodically, at regular intervals.

REVIEW QUESTIONS

1. Define the terms 'Accreditation' and 'NABL'.
2. Write a note on NABL Accreditation and its advantages.
3. List out the steps for NABL accreditation in India.
4. Describe how a laboratory must prepare for NABL accreditation.

🖎 🖎 🖎

Chapter ... **7**

ORGANIZATION AND PERSONNEL

Objectives:

Upon completion of this section, the student should be able to

- List out the responsibilities of key personnel in a pharmaceutical manufacturing unit.
- Describe functions of the Quality Control (QC) unit.
- Explain the education, training and other requirements for personnel in the organization.
- Outline the health and hygiene requirements for personnel.

Introduction

In the complex field of pharmaceutical manufacturing, it is important to have a sound quality system in place to make sure that products manufactured have the desired quality, safety and efficacy. At the same time, it is vital to recognize that even the best quality system is only as good as the people who make it work. Personnel are the backbone of the manufacturing unit, and there must be a sufficient number of adequately qualified and trained staff to ensure one achieves the desired quality products. No person should be so burdened with responsibilities that it presents a quality risk.

7.1 ORGANIZATION

Sufficient number of personnel must be present to perform as well as to supervise the manufacture, processing, packing and holding of every drug product. In any pharma unit, it is important to lay out individual responsibilities in a manner that is clear enough to be understood by the personnel who are to perform the respective tasks. Written job descriptions must be available and an organization chart must be prepared to show the hierarchical organization of employees.

Responsibilities of Key Personnel

Production Head responsibilities	Quality Control Head responsibilities	Shared responsibilities
Production and storage of products as per requirements.	Approval or rejection of starting materials, intermediate and finished products and packaging materials.	Monitoring and approval of material suppliers and contract manufacturers.

... (Contd.)

Production Head responsibilities	Quality Control Head responsibilities	Shared responsibilities
Approval of instructions for processing operations.	Evaluation of batch records.	Monitoring and control of environment in the production areas.
Evaluation and signing of production records.	Approval of specifications, test methods, sampling methods and other QC procedures.	Ensuring validations are carried out.
Verification of maintenance of premises, equipment and manufacturing and packing areas.	Ensuring testing is performed as per protocols.	Training of personnel.
Ensure periodic personnel training is performed.	Monitoring and approval of contract analysis.	Monitoring compliance with cGMPs.

7.2 RESPONSIBILITIES OF QC UNIT

Every pharmaceutical manufacturing unit should have a quality control unit. There must be written procedures to describe the functioning and responsibilities of this unit, and these procedures must be followed.

The QC unit has the responsibility of testing all raw materials, drug products, containers, closures, in-process materials, labeling and packaging material. It also has the authority to accordingly approve the materials that meet quality, safety and efficacy specifications and reject the ones that do not meet them.

The QC unit also has the authority to review the records generated during production of every batch to ensure that errors have not occurred at any stage or that any errors that occurred have been completely investigated. In case a company A gets products manufactured under contract by another company B, the QC unit of A has the authority to approve or reject those products manufactured, packed, processed or held by B for A.

The QC unit must have access to necessary laboratory space and facilities to test and approve all raw materials, drug products, containers, closures, in-process materials, labeling and packaging material.

Any procedures or specifications that are likely to impact the strength, identity, purity and quality of the drug product must be approved by the QC unit.

7.3 PERSONNEL RESPONSIBILITIES

All persons involved with the manufacture, processing, packing or holding of drug products must wear clothing that is clean and suitable for the work to be performed. Wherever required, personnel must wear adequate protective apparel to cover their face, hands, arms, head etc to prevent contamination of the drug product.

Personnel must practice good health and sanitation habits. They must enter only those areas of the premises that they have been authorized to enter. Limited access areas can be entered only after due authorization by the supervisory persons.

7.4 PERSONNEL QUALIFICATIONS

All persons engaged in the manufacturing, processing, packing or holding of drug products must have the necessary education, training and experience, or an acceptable combination of these to ensure they are capable of carrying out the assigned work.

Personnel must be trained on the particular operations they perform and on the current Good Manufacturing Practices (cGMP) that are relevant to their area of work. cGMP training must be imparted on a regular basis by adequately qualified trainers to ensure the employees stay current in their information about the relevant cGMP requirements.

Every person who supervises the manufacture, processing, packing or holding of drug products must have the necessary education, training and experience, or an acceptable combination of these to ensure they are capable of carrying out the assigned supervisory work.

7.5 KEY PERSONNEL

Key positions must be held by full-time personnel. This generally includes the heads of production and quality control and the authorized person. The heads of quality control and production must be independent of each other and they bear the responsibility of all actions performed by their subordinates. The key personnel must have sufficient scientific education and practical experience in the manufacture of drug products in keeping with national regulatory guidelines. They must be capable of making independent judgment based on applying scientific thought to the problems that may be encountered while performing their responsibilities.

The authorized person is responsible to implement the quality system, perform internal audit or self inspection, and participate in validation programs. This person is ultimately held accountable for any non-compliance with regulatory requirements.

7.6 PERSONNEL TRAINING

All personnel entering the manufacturing areas and quality control laboratories (including housekeeping staff) must be trained according to a written program. The training programs must cover technical aspects of their work, and also the theory and practice of cGMP. Personnel working in clean areas or areas where hazardous materials are being handled must be imparted specific training on the precautions they must follow to avoid contaminating the product or the environment and also for personal safety. Training must be done at regular intervals and the effectiveness of the training must be assessed. Records of personnel training must be maintained.

7.7 PERSONNEL HEALTH AND HYGIENE

Personnel to be employed in a drug product manufacturing facility must undergo health examination before being hired. Only those who are free from contagious, communicable conditions, skin diseases and tuberculosis must be given employment. Persons to be employed in an area where beta lactam antibiotics are being manufactured must be tested for sensitivity to penicillin before being employed.

Those employees who need to perform visual inspections must have periodic eye checkups. Personnel handling cytotoxic drugs, sex hormones and other potent medicaments must be examined regularly for any adverse effect of these substances. As a safety measure, it is good to rotate staff in these special areas.

Personnel must be trained in personal hygiene aspects such as washing their hands, donning appropriate protective clothing, using a face mask and hair cap etc before entering manufacturing areas. Change rooms must be provided with facilities for storing personal belongings, and ensuring personal hygiene (wash basins, running water, hand dryers, disinfectants etc).

Employees must be instructed about not allowing direct contact between their hands and any raw material, in-process goods or finished, unpacked drug product.

If any person is found to have an open lesion or an illness (by observation of the supervisor or through a medical examination) that may have an impact on the quality or safety of drug products, that person must be kept away from coming into direct contact with drug product, containers and closures and in-process materials until declared fit to do so by a medical professional. Personnel must be instructed to themselves report any such medical conditions to their supervisors.

Personnel must not be allowed to eat, drink, smoke or chew anything in the production, laboratory and storage areas.

A team of skilled and trained personnel is one of the biggest factors that influence the production of quality products that are safe and efficacious. Ultimately, it is the people handling the process who will decide its success. When personnel understand their responsibilities, get trained on cGMP and perform their tasks in keeping with the SOPs, it ensures that the product quality will be of the desired level and meet the predetermined specifications.

REVIEW QUESTIONS

1. Explain the division of responsibilities between the Production and QC Heads in a pharma company.

2. Describe the types of training that must be given to personnel in a pharmaceutical unit.

3. What precautions must be taken from the health and hygiene point of personnel?

Chapter ...**8**

PREMISES - DESIGN, CONSTRUCTION, LAYOUT AND MAINTENANCE

Objectives:

Upon completion of this section, the student should be able to

- List important factors in deciding on the location of a pharmaceutical manufacturing unit.
- Describe important utilities in a manufacturing plant.
- Outline the need for sanitation and how it is to be achieved.
- Define the clean room requirements as per different regulatory bodies.
- Explain the dangers of cross contamination and how to avoid these.
- Describe specific requirements for different areas in the pharmaceutical plant.

Introduction

In any industry, manufacturing operations must be carried out under clean and hygienic conditions. However, in the pharmaceutical industry, the condition of the premises assumes critical importance because of the nature of the products being manufactured. Both the external and internal environments must be geared to be conducive to maintain the quality and safety of drug products. Special care must also be taken to prevent contamination of the products and therefore, the location, design, construction and layout of premises is a vital part of the Good Manufacturing Practices (GMP) regulations. 'Premises' refers to the buildings and facilities where pharmaceutical processing is done. These places must comply with cGMP requirements.

8.1 LOCATION

Premises must be located in a site that is of a size suitable to house all the different departments. The nature of manufacturing and testing to be performed, the magnitude of the operation in terms of daily production levels, the number of products that will be processed and the storage space required for raw material, in-process and finished goods are some of the important factors to be considered when choosing a location. Other factors such as availability of power, water, labour workforce and closeness to transport hubs may also impact this decision. From the GMP point of view, the most important factor is the climatic condition, and hygiene levels in the surroundings. Pharmaceutical premises must ideally be located away from polluting industries as otherwise, it will burden the air handling and water handling systems.

According to Schedule M of the Drugs and Cosmetics Rules, factory buildings must be situated in a place that avoids contamination risk from the external environment (for example – from open drains, public lavatory, open sewage lines, or industry that produces gaseous fumes or strong odours or generates smoke, dust or other chemical emissions).

8.2 DESIGN AND CONSTRUCTION

The building used must be designed, constructed and maintained in a manner that permits drug production under hygienic conditions. It must be suitable for the operations being performed. The layout of the premises must be such that it reduces risk of errors, and also avoids buildup of dirt and cross-contamination that may affect drug product quality. Construction and layout of the building must allow for a sequential and logical flow of the production process and movement of personnel and materials. It must also permit regular cleaning, repair and maintenance work without harming product quality.

Walls, ceilings and floors of the building must be smooth and crack-free, easy to clean and disinfect. Surfaces must not shed particles; they must be kept smooth and without any open joints where dust can accumulate.

8.3 UTILITIES

The building must be supplied with adequate light, water, power supply and ventilation and must be fitted with systems to maintain the temperature and humidity of different areas at desired levels. There must be arrangements to protect against the entry of pests, insects, rodents etc.

The fittings, ducts, pipes and ventilation points must be designed in such a way that they do not produce difficult-to-clean recesses. Such points must be located to be easily accessible for maintenance work without having to enter the manufacturing areas.

Sensitive drug manufacturing areas must be air-conditioned to achieve the optimum temperature and humidity conditions. All areas must receive filtered air – the filtration and air change rate must be designed to achieve the desired clean area classification. Some of the important factors that influence this rate include the quality of the input air, size of the room, heat load of the room, room pressure to be maintained, dust generated during processing in that room, number of personnel working in the room etc. An air change rate of 6 to 20 air changes per hour is the norm.

Lighting facilities too must match requirements – for example, visual inspection areas must be brightly lit; light-sensitive drug manufacturing requires amber lighting provisions etc.

Water systems shall be installed to provide water of the quality commensurate with requirements of the drug product. Potable water may be used for washing and cleaning but better quality water as purified water or distilled water must be used during the manufacturing and testing operations. Water storage tanks must be designed to maintain the quality of the water and prevent microbial growth.

8.4 SANITATION

All areas inside the building must be cleaned regularly and cleaning records must be maintained. Drains must be sized correctly and be designed to prevent back-flow of contents. They must be closed as far as possible; if open channels are unavoidable, they must be kept shallow to allow easy cleaning and disinfection.

Wastes from manufacturing area must be disposed in keeping with regulations of Environment Pollution Control Board. Waste materials that have to be disposed must be stored in a safe manner. Any wastes that are inflammable, hazardous or toxic must be stored in a segregated area while awaiting disposal. Bio-medical waste must be disposed as per regulations of Bio-Medical Waste (Management and Handling) Rules, 1996. Rejected drugs must be stored separately and destroyed in keeping with regulations.

Restrooms, toilets and refreshment area must be located far from manufacturing areas. They must not be in direct communication with areas where materials are manufactured, tested or stored. Animal testing laboratories too must be isolated from these areas, with separate entrance and dedicated air-handling systems.

8.4.1 Sanitation of Sterile Areas

Sterile areas must be cleaned and sanitized often in keeping with an approved cleaning protocol. More than one type of disinfectants must be used to ensure effective bactericidal action. Regular monitoring of clean rooms must be performed to detect presence of contaminating microorganisms. Cleaning procedures must be validated to verify that disinfectant residues are detected and removed during cleaning. Detergents and disinfectants used in sterile areas must be sterile before use. For spaces that are inaccessible inside the sterile room, fumigation may be used to reduce microbial contamination. Occasional cleaning with a sporicidal agent must be part of the cleaning routine since spores are resistant to the common disinfectants.

8.5 ENVIRONMENTAL CONTROL

The temperature and relative humidity of the premises must be controlled in order to ensure the area complies with material and product requirements, as well as regulatory requirements. Attention must also be given to operator comfort wherever possible. Airlocks must be built to separate low-humidity areas from higher humidity areas; this prevents the migration of moisture that would otherwise overload the Heating Ventilation and Air Conditioning (HVAC) system.

The systems used for humidity control must be designed to avoid introducing any contaminants.

Dust and vapours must be extracted at source and not allowed to travel elsewhere. The dust extraction system must have adequate transfer velocity in order to make sure that the dust is truly carried away and does not merely settle into the ducting of the system.

General direction of airflow in a room must be designed to remove vapours and dust generated in the area. It must also consider the location of the operator to make sure he/she does not contribute to contamination. It is often preferred to introduce air into the room using ceiling diffusers, and extract the room air through vents at low heights on the wall to provide a flushing effect as the air moves out of the room. In case of processes that generate a vapor that is lighter than air, the extraction grilles will need to be positioned at higher level.

8.6 CONTAMINATION

World Health Organization (WHO) defines contamination as, "The undesired introduction of impurities of a chemical or microbial nature, or of foreign matter, into or on to a starting material or intermediate, during production, sampling, packaging or repackaging, storage or transport."

The most common sources of contamination are dust, skin, hair, microorganisms, grease, chemicals and particulate matter. Such contamination can be controlled by controlling the environmental conditions as well as personnel factors.

Environment control is exerted by having a well-designed HVAC system that efficiently removes the contaminants that may get introduced. Regular cleaning and controlled entry and exit of materials and personnel into the clean areas can also help avoid contamination.

Personnel hygiene is a must and they must be trained to follow the prescribed dress code, procedures for entry and exit into clean rooms and gowning procedures.

Cleanrooms:

Cleanroom refers to a controlled environment where level of contamination is kept very low to meet requirements specified in terms of number of particulates per cubic meter. To achieve this controlled environment, air enters the cleanroom through High Efficiency Particulate Air (HEPA) filters that remove particles greater than or equal to 0.3 micron in size.

US Food and Drug Administration Guideline for Air Classification

			Microbiological Limit	
Clean area classification	**0.5 µm particles /ft^3**	**0.5 µm particles /mt^3**	**cfu/ ft^3**	**cfu/ mt^3**
100	100	3500	< 1	< 3
1000	1000	35000	< 2	< 7
10000	10000	350000	< 3	< 18
100000	100000	3500000	< 25	< 88
Note : µm – micrometer, ft^3 – cubic feet, mt^3 – cubic meter, cfu – colony forming unit				

Cleanroom Classification as per Schedule M:

Grade	At rest (b)		In operation (a)	
	Maximum number of permitted particles per cubic metre equal to or above			
	0.5 µm	5 µm	0.5 µm	5 µm
A	3520	29	3500	29
B (a)	35,200	293	3,52,000	2,930
C (a)	3,52,000	2,930	35,20,000	29,300
D (a)	35,20,000	29,300	Not defined (c)	Not defined (c)

Grade	Types of operations for aseptic preparations
A	Aseptic preparations and filling.
B	Background room conditions for activities requiring Grade A.
C	Preparation of solution to be filtered.
D	Handling of components after washing.

WHO Air Classification System for Manufacture of Sterile Products

Grade	Maximum number of particle permitted per m^3		Maximum number of viable microorganisms per m^3
	0.5 – 5 µm	> 5 µm	
A (Laminar airflow workstation)	3,500	None	Less than 1
B	3,500	None	5
C	3,50,000	2000	100
D	35,00,000	20,000	500

8.7 CROSS CONTAMINATION

WHO defines cross-contamination as, "Contamination of a starting material, intermediate product or a finished product with another starting material or material during production."

Manufacturing areas must be designed to prevent both contamination of drug product and cross contamination between products. Contamination may be avoided by controlling the quality of air in a room and by ensuring hygiene and clothing change of workers entering into the manufacturing area. Cross-contamination is a little more difficult to control.

Risk of cross-contamination is greater when dry material processing takes place because dust is generated and spreads rapidly. The most common sources of cross-contamination include dust, vapors, gases, particles, sprays, residues on equipment surfaces, operators clothing or skin.

The most dangerous contaminants include sensitizing materials, hormones, living organisms, cytotoxic materials and highly active compounds.

8.7.1 Measures to Prevent/ Reduce Cross-contamination

1. Manufacturing the product in dedicated areas which are self-contained.
2. Manufacturing on a campaign basis – complete the production process and then ensure a thorough cleaning before starting a new product batch on the same line.
3. Using premises that are appropriately protected through airlocks, air-extraction systems and pressure differentials.
4. Preventing re-entry or re-circulation of untreated air.
5. Using protective clothing.
6. Regular testing for presence of residues.

8.7.2 Preventing Dust Migration in Non-dedicated Facilities

Sometimes, it may be necessary to manufacture different products in different areas of the same premises. In such situations, care must be taken to ensure dust from one area doesn't move into another area where a different product is being processed.

8.7.3 Air Containment

Containment of air is achieved by two methods – displacement or pressure differential.

Displacement Concept:

This concept relies on maintaining a high airflow in combination with a low pressure differential. It is often used in areas where dust generation is high. Air is supplied into the corridor, from where it flows through the doorway and into the room, and gets extracted out from the back of the room. The room door must be kept closed and air entry is through a door grille. The air should move with a velocity that's high enough to ensure there is no turbulence in the doorway that may cause dust to escape.

Pressure Differential Concept:

This relies on use of low airflow in combination with a high pressure differential. This concept works best in areas that are no-dust or low-dust. The pressure differential between clean and less-clean areas must be great enough to ensure air containment and prevent reverse-flow of air; however, it must not be high enough to cause turbulence in the area. Generally, pressure differentials of 5Pa to 20 Pa are acceptable; the most commonly maintained value is 15 Pa. Too low pressure differentials must be avoided because they lead to reversal of air flow, and contamination. If unavoidable, it is advised to simultaneously use airlocks too.

These areas must be fitted with devices to control and monitoring devices that must be qualified before use. Regular calibration of these devices is also necessary. There must also be an alarm system linked to the pressure controller to alert personnel to any critical change in the pressure differentials.

8.7.4 Airlocks

The barrier which separates two controlled areas is called as an airlock. It generally has two or more doors to regulate the movement of air. Airlocks can be of three types – cascade type, bubble type and sink type.

(a) Cascade airlocks: These airlocks have lower pressure on one side, and higher pressure on the other side. For example, in tablet manufacturing areas, corridor is at higher pressure, and cubicle where drug processing occurs is at lower pressure. Thus, air moves from corridor to cubicle, and prevents dust containing drug from entering into the corridor.

(b) Bubble airlocks: These airlocks have higher pressure inside than on both outer sides. For example, in parenteral manufacturing areas, the high pressure inside drives air away from the room into the corridor. Thus, entry of contaminants that may damage the drug inside the sterile clean room is prevented.

(c) Sink airlocks: Here, the pressure on both sides of the airlock is very high so that no contaminant can escape from the cubicle. This type of system is used in facilities used to manufacture harmful substances like toxins or poisons.

In all these airlocks, doors must open into the side having higher pressure so that it will close automatically and faster. The airlock must be designed with an interlocking system so that both doors cannot open at the same time. Opening of either door must be linked to the sounding of an alarm.

Air changes must be carried out at higher rates within the airlock – generally, 20 air changes per hour is the minimum prescribed rate. Airlocks must be empty; no material should be stored in them.

8.8 ADDITIONAL CONSIDERATIONS REGARDING PREMISES

8.8.1 Storage Areas

Storage areas must have sufficient space for the materials to be stored in a systematic and organized manner according to their categories such as starting materials, intermediates, bulk product, finished products, packaging materials, released products, quarantined products, rejected products, recalled products and returned products.

These areas must be clean, well-lit, dry, and be maintained at specified temperatures. In case of special storage conditions (for example, cold conditions), the conditions must be monitored and controlled.

Receiving bays must allow cleaning of incoming material if necessary. The received material must be kept in quarantine until sampling, testing and approval. Entry to this area must be restricted. Materials that have been rejected or returned or recalled must be physically separated from other materials. Separate storage areas must exist for holding materials that are dangerous or highly active (for example – narcotics, highly inflammable solvents, radioactive materials, poisons etc.).

Sampling areas for starting materials must be sufficiently separated to avoid contamination or cross contamination.

8.8.2 Production Areas

Products that are highly active (such as hormones, antibiotics, cytotoxic drugs) or highly sensitizing (penicillin, for example) must be manufactured in dedicated facilities that are self-contained. Other products must not be manufactured here.

In facilities where multiple product batches are being simultaneously manufactured, there must be measures in place to prevent cross-contamination. Besides, there must be sufficient in-process storage space to prevent the occurrence of mix-ups.

8.8.3 Quality Control (QC) Laboratory Areas

QC laboratories must be located in an area separate from production. In the laboratories, separate areas must exist for biological, microbiological, and radioisotope testing and these areas must have dedicated air handling units. Sufficient space must be provided for storing samples, solvents, reference standards and laboratory records with no chances of mix-ups between different samples drawn for testing. Air supply to QC laboratories must be separate from the unit supplying air to production areas.

Instruments that are sensitive to temperature and humidity must be housed in separate rooms. Care must be taken to prevent vibrations and electrical interference from reaching them.

Pharmaceutical companies pay lot of attention to setting up quality management systems and validation studies in order to ensure regulatory compliance. Along with this, it is vital they pay attention to maintenance of their facilities and premises so that there is no risk of product contamination which may lead to damaging situations such a s a product recall. Having self-inspection programmes, regular maintenance activity, and good housekeeping practices will ensure that companies remain in compliance with regulatory requirements.

REVIEW QUESTIONS

1. List out the factors to be considered when deciding where to set up a pharmaceutical plant.

2. What are the important sanitation and utility requirements for pharmaceutical manufacturing areas?

3. Explain the different classifications of clean rooms as per the guidelines of USFDA and Schedule M.

4. Define airlocks. Explain different types and how they work.

5. Discuss the measures to be taken to maintain the environment of a pharmaceutical manufacturing plant.

Chapter ...9

EQUIPMENTS AND RAW MATERIALS

Objectives:

Upon completion of this section, the student should be able to

- Outline the importance of equipment design and location.
- List the important factors considered while selecting equipment for purchase.
- Describe the measures to be taken in raw material purchase, receiving, storage and handling.
- Define the different labels used in raw material handling.
- Explain the sampling, testing and handling of raw materials.

9.1 EQUIPMENTS

The pharmaceutical industry makes use of different equipment at each stage of the manufacturing of drug products. Equipment used may be a single piece – such as a weighing machine, or a granulator – or a group of equipment working in a process to deliver a single outcome – such as a purified water system.

The ingredients of a formulation come into intimate contact with the equipment at every step. Naturally, the quality of this equipment plays a major role in determining the quality of the final products. Equipment must be designed and constructed in a manner that prevents contamination or any other adverse impact on the drug material.

9.1.1 Design and Construction

Equipment must be designed and constructed to suit the purpose of its use. The material of construction must be adequate to the nature of processing to be undertaken. Equipment surfaces that come into contact with drug product must not be additive, reactive or absorptive. If the surface of equipment adds chemicals from its surface into the drug material, or reacts with it or absorbs the formulation ingredients, there can be a serious impact on the identity, safety, strength, purity and quality of the final product.

Equipment must be designed for closed operation as far as possible to reduce the risk of contamination of material it holds. If open equipment is unavoidable, it must be designed and handled in a way that minimizes contamination. Diagrams of critical equipment must be maintained. Lubricants used in equipment maintenance should be of non-toxic or edible grade. Such lubricants or coolants used on the equipment must not come into contact with the drug product, its containers or closures. Failure to ensure this will contaminate the drug and render it unsafe for use.

9.1.2 Location

Equipment must be located in a clean, hygienic area that is suitable for the operation being performed. When several equipments are to be used as part of a process, they must be located in such a way as to allow the linear and sequential flow of the production process. The equipment must be situated in a way that it allows ease of cleaning and maintenance.

9.1.3 Installation

Equipment must be installed in keeping with the manufacturer's specifications. All necessary utilities must be provided and there must be arrangements to access the equipment for maintenance work without having to enter the production areas. Pipework leading to and from any equipment must be labeled with contents and direction of flow. Any equipment that is defective must be removed to a separate area outside the production or quality control area. In case this is not possible, the equipment must bear a conspicuous label that states its defective status.

9.1.4 Cleaning and Maintenance

Written procedures must exist for the cleaning of equipment and their regular maintenance. Cleaning must be done at regular intervals to avoid the entry of contaminants; equipment must also be cleaned thoroughly between different batches of product to avoid risk of cross-contamination. For equipment used in manufacturing sterile products, additional steps need to be taken to sanitize and sterilize the equipment to maintain it in sterile condition. Regular maintenance must be performed for all critical equipment to ensure there are no malfunctions during a processing run. Cleaning validation studies must be performed to ensure equipment cleaning leads to the desired levels of cleanliness.

9.1.5 Qualification and Calibration

Qualification of equipment begins right at the design state when it is designed to be constructed in a particular manner suitable to its intended purpose. Steps of design qualification (DQ), installation qualification (IQ), operational qualification (OQ) and performance qualification (PQ) must be carried out to ensure the equipment is designed, installed, operated and performed as expected to give a quality product.

Once equipment has become operational, with wear and tear over time, there is a chance of a drift in its performance from expected profiles. So, it is vital to have a regular calibration program in which the equipment and any associated instruments are checked to obtain a measure of how accurately it is performing. These calibration results can help to identify defects in the equipment, which can then be dealt with in the appropriate manner.

Records of calibration and qualification must be maintained for all equipment.

When computer or related systems are used, there must be sufficient control to ensure that any changes in records take place only after due authorization by higher management. Backup files of data must be maintained and stored in a way that it is protected from alteration or loss. Hard copies of backup data must be maintained, too.

9.1.6 Documentation

All the major equipments should have a unique identification code or number, and this must be recorded in the batch manufacturing record (BMR). Separate cleaning and maintenance logs must be maintained for each of the major equipment, and any cleaning or maintenance activity must be recorded in these. Standard operating procedures must exist for operating all equipment, and they must be placed close to the equipment for use by the personnel handling them.

The major equipment being used in manufacturing a given batch must be labeled with details of product name and batch number at all times to indicate the contents within.

9.1.7 Purchase Specifications for Equipment

Pharmaceutical industry equipment is quite expensive and therefore, selecting the right equipment is a critical process. Some of the most important factors to be considered in making this decision are as follows:

- **Desired output capacity:** Equipment purchased must be capable of processing desired quantity of product at the desired speed of operation. Understanding one's production scale in terms of batch size requirements and comparing this with the load capacity of the equipment being considered is an important first step when choosing equipment.

- **Product characteristics:** The nature of the product, its reactivity, any special conditions necessary to ensure retention of its safety, efficacy and quality are all important while choosing equipment.

- **Ease of operation:** Equipment operation must be simple, and not involve complex maneuvers or require special skills. The equipment must be easy for the operator to operate after receiving proper training. It is important to strike a balance between efficiency of performing the given operation and ease of operating the equipment. Digitally enabled equipment can help to manage manufacturing process better; it will however require special skills for operation and the capacity of one's workforce to learn those skills must be considered.

- **Ease of cleaning and maintenance:** Equipment will require regular cleaning and special, more thorough cleaning between batches of different products. The time used for cleaning is time lost from the production run. So equipment must be easy to clean (either in-place, or by disconnecting and taking to a special cleaning area). It must also be easy to maintain and not require frequent maintenance activities which again are a time-consuming process.

- **Equipment supplier:** When buying equipment, price is often considered an important criterion, but it is more important to focus on the quality parameters on offer and the industry reputation of the supplier and how reliable their product is, their customer service, and their capability to provide equipment troubleshooting service when necessary.

9.2 RAW MATERIAL

Between 1995 and 1996, Haiti saw incidents of around 80 children dying after ingesting a cold-and-cough syrup. An investigation fixed the responsibility on glycerol in the product being contaminated with diethylene glycol. This and other such incidents highlight the need for drug product manufacturers to pay attention to the quality of starting materials they use.

While active pharmaceutical ingredients (APIs) may be manufactured under cGMP (current Good Manufacturing Practices), excipients may not be so produced, especially the ones commonly used in other industries like cosmetics or food. This makes it even more important to ensure these excipients are of a grade suitable for pharmaceutical use. Containers and closures must also be evaluated because they play a vital role in ensuring product stays stable and safe throughout the shelf life.

9.2.1 Purchase of Materials

Purchasing must be done by staff with a thorough knowledge of those materials and their suppliers. Materials must be procured only from approved suppliers who have consented to provide materials in keeping with quality specifications of the drug product manufacturer. It is advisable for pharmaceutical manufacturer's to enter into contracts with specific vendors after performing a vendor audit that provides an assurance of raw materials and packaging materials of the desired level of safety and meeting quality standards.

9.2.3 Receiving, handling and storage of materials

Specific written procedures must be prepared to describe how materials (both drug components and drug containers and closures) will be received, identified, stored, handled, sampled, tested and accordingly approved or rejected, and these procedures must be followed as written.

When receiving materials, the consignment must be visually examined and the labels checked to confirm the content, quantity, integrity of seals and to verify that there is no damage or contamination. Any damaged containers found must be separated, and details recorded and informed to the supplier.

The materials must be stored under quarantine until samples have been drawn and tests have been performed. They must not be issued for use before approval.

Handling and storage of all materials in the storage area must be in such a way that there is no contamination. Boxes or bags holding containers and closures must be stored off the floor. The storage must be done in a way that suitable space is left for proper cleaning and inspection of the materials.

9.2.4 Sampling

Representative samples must be drawn from each shipment of each lot. If different batches are present in a single shipment, samples must be drawn from each of those. The quantity must be sufficient to perform all required tests and reserve when specified. Statistical criteria must also be used to determine quantity of samples drawn. Containers must be cleaned before sampling to avoid introducing contamination, and resealed after sampling to prevent contamination of the contents, and appropriately labeled to show sample has been taken. Samples must be drawn from the bottom, middle and top of the containers, and marked accordingly. Sample-holding containers shall be labeled with details of name of material, lot number, container number, date of sampling, and name of person collecting the sample.

9.2.5 Testing of Samples

At least one specific test must be performed to verify the material's identity. Tests must be carried out to determine conformity with predetermined specifications for quality, strength and purity. In case materials are supplied along with a certificate of analysis by the supplier, the materials may be used without sampling and testing, provided the supplier is a reliable, validated vendor and at least one specific identity test has been performed and mentioned in the certificate.

Materials that are liable to contamination with adulterants, or insect infestations or filth must be examined for such contaminants. If materials are prone to microbial contamination, microbiological tests must be performed to test for it.

9.2.6 Approval/Rejection of Materials

All materials that meet the manufacturer's quality requirements of identity, quality, purity and strength and other tests are to be approved for use. Materials not meeting these requirements must be rejected.

9.2.7 Labeling

Labels must carry the name of the product, the company's unique reference code, manufacturer's name and address, and their assigned batch number. It must also state the status of the contents (For example – "Sampled", "Quarantined", "Approved" and "Rejected"), manufacturing and expiry dates and re-test date. When attaching such labels, care must be taken that original information on the supplier's label is not lost.

Approved materials must be so marked while rejected materials must be conspicuously labeled and stored in a separate area to avoid chances of mix-ups or misuse.

9.2.8 Using Approved Materials

Approved materials must be stored properly and issued for use in a way such that earliest approved stock is used first before more recently approved stock. Many companies use a FEFO (First Expire First Out) system for stock rotation. Another deciding factor is that the drug product's shelf life must not exceed the shelf life of the APIs.

If materials have been stored for very long period without usage, or if they have been exposed to any condition that may have an adverse effect on their quality or safety, they must be re-tested for the same parameters as the initial test. Results of the re-test must be used to determine if the materials are approved or rejected.

9.2.9 Handling Rejected Materials

Rejected materials must be identified with appropriate labels and kept in quarantine until safely disposed. Care must be taken to prevent use of such materials in manufacturing operations.

9.2.10 Containers and Closures

Containers and closures are used for packing of drug products must not be additive, reactive or absorptive. This is important to ensure they do not cause a change in the identity, safety, quality, strength, or purity of the drugs beyond specifications.

Closures and containers must be capable of protecting the drug product from external conditions that may cause its contamination or deterioration.

Containers and closures must be clean and if required, sterilized to remove contamination by microorganisms and pyrogens.

Note: If computerized storage systems are used, they must be fully validated to prove they work reliably.

REVIEW QUESTIONS

1. List out the important factors to be considered in equipment design and location.
2. Name and explain the 3 most important criteria that matter when purchasing equipment.
3. Describe the procedures followed for sampling and testing of raw materials.
4. Write a note on labelling of raw materials.
5. Explain the steps in the approval/rejection of raw materials by the QC department.

✍ ✍ ✍

Chapter ...**10**

QUALITY CONTROL

Objectives:

Upon completion of this section, the student should be able to

- Define Quality Control (QC) in pharmaceutical industry and its scope.
- Outline the organization of the QC unit.
- Explain the responsibilities of the QC unit.
- Define and explain the concept of Out Of Specification (OOS) results.
- Describe the investigation of OOS results.
- List important functions of packaging.
- Classify packaging materials in the pharmaceutical industry.
- Describe important QC tests for packaging materials.
- Explain specific pharmacopoeial tests for containers, closures and secondary packing materials.

Introduction

Along with safety and efficacy, quality is one of the most important criteria to assess the fitness of a medicinal product for use by the patient. This parameter is not something that can be achieved by itself, without any effort. While the earlier concept was to test products for quality, the pharmaceutical industry has now moved on to building quality into products right from the design stage itself. However, quality control (QC) still plays a vital role in giving a high degree of assurance that products are meeting their specifications.

10.1 DEFINITION

10.1.1 WHO

The World Health Organization (WHO) defines the term quality control as, "The sum of all procedures undertaken to ensure the identity and purity of a particular pharmaceutical. Such procedures may range from the performance of simple chemical experiments which determine the identity and screening for the presence of particular pharmaceutical substance (thin layer chromatography, infrared spectroscopy etc.), to more complicated requirements of pharmacopoeial monographs."

10.1.2 Schedule M

Schedule M of the Indian Drugs and Cosmetics Act and Rules defines a QC system as follows:

"Quality Control shall be concerned with sampling, specifications, testing, documentation, release procedures which ensure that the necessary and relevant tests are actually carried and that the materials are not released for use, nor products released for sale or supply until their quality has been judged to be satisfactory. It is not confined to laboratory operations but shall be involved in all decisions concerning the quality of the product. It shall be ensured that all quality control arrangements are effectively and reliably carried out the department as a whole shall have other duties such as to establish evaluate, validate and implement all Quality Control Procedures and methods."

10.2 SCOPE OF QC

Pharmaceutical QC aims at investigating manufactured drug products according to compendial specifications and standards to monitor that they are of the required quality. QC is concerned with setting up specifications, drawing samples, testing them and generating documentation related to the tests and their reports. QC also evaluates the analysis reports and ensures that no material is released for use or for supply or sale until it meets the necessary quality requirements and pre-determined specifications. The scope of QC is not limited to mere laboratory work; this department is involved in all situations that involve quality of the product.

10.3 ORGANIZATION OF QC

Drug manufacturers are required to set up their own QC labs and employ staff with the necessary qualifications and training to perform the necessary tests. The department must have adequate space to perform all the analyses, store data related to them, and also store reference samples from each batch of product shipped from the company.

Most quality control laboratories are divided into different types of testing – chemical, instrumental, biological and microbiological.

One of the fundamental requirements for the QC department is that it must be independent of all the other departments. The QC Head must report directly to the topmost authority, and not to the Production Head.

10.4 RESPONSIBILITIES OF QC

Responsibilities of QC are as follows :

1. Preparing specifications for all raw materials, packing materials, finished products, intermediates and solvents and reagents used in analyses.

2. Inspecting, sampling and testing of all starting materials including packaging materials, intermediate and finished products as per procedures defined in the Standard Operating Procedures (SOPs).

3. Performing stability testing to assess product stability.

4. Monitoring environmental conditions are met as per current Good Manufacturing Practices (cGMP) requirements.

5. Preparing analysis reports for the tested samples, and recording and investigation any results that are Out Of Specifications (OOS).

6. Approving product batches for sale after ensuring it meets quality, safety and efficacy standards prescribed.

7. Calibration of all laboratory instruments and devices used in the testing.

8. Validation of analytical methods used in the testing.

9. Retaining reference samples from each batch of product released to the market.

10. Reviewing the batch manufacturing and packing records and assessing the test reports to ensure products are of the desired quality and have been properly packed and labeled.

11. Participating in any investigation that follows market complaints about the quality of a product.

10.5 SAMPLING

QC personnel must be authorized to enter the stores and production areas for sampling of materials, intermediates and final products. The samples must be drawn in keeping with approved written procedures in a way to be truly representative of the materials. Care must be taken during sampling to avoid contamination of the containers, and also the mix-up of materials sampled. This is achieved by using clean and sterilized (if necessary) sampling equipment.

The containers from which samples have been drawn must be resealed correctly after sampling. Such containers must be labeled with details of name of material, batch or lot number, sampling date, and signature of the sampler.

10.6 TESTING AND ANALYSIS

Analysis must be performed on the samples drawn, and results informed to the stores and production heads. Containers must duly be affixed with "Approved" or "Rejected" labels as the case may be; rejected material must be removed to a separate area with entry restricted to authorized persons only.

10.7 PRODUCT ASSESSMENT

All batch processing records must be reviewed for conditions under which production was done and results of testing of starting material, in-process and finished products must be studied. Compliance of final product to specifications and presence of complete documentation must be confirmed. After verifying all these, the assessment records are signed by the Production Head and the QC Head and only then is the product released for distribution and sale.

10.8 REFERENCE SAMPLES/RETAINED SAMPLES

Samples must be retained from every batch of product released to the market. Quantity of these retained samples must be at least double the quantity required to conduct all tests. They must be retained in their final packs for a duration of 3 months after their expiry date. If any market complaints are received following supply and sale, the reference samples must be examined and analyzed to determine veracity of the complaint.

10.9 OUT OF SPECIFICATIONS (OOS) RESULTS

According to United States Food and Drug Administration (USFDA), OOS results are defined as, "All test results that fall outside the specifications or acceptance criteria established in drug applications, drug master files (DMFs), official compendia, or by the manufacturer. The term also applies to all in-process laboratory tests that are outside of established specifications."

OOS results indicate a loss of control over either the manufacturing or the analytical process, or both. This can result in defective products being sent out, and subsequent market complaints or product recalls, and even a threat to life of the patients. So, it is vital to investigate OOS results and identify and address the root causes responsible for the OOS result.

There must be written and approved procedures to investigate any OOS results and these must be followed. OOS result investigation generally proceeds in two phases.

Phase I: Laboratory Investigation

Here, the objective is to identify the cause of the OOS result. It may arise from an aberration in either the analytical process or the manufacturing process. If OOS result causes rejection of a batch of product, it is still necessary to investigate the cause, and check if there may have been an impact on any other batch of same or different products.

In this phase, the accuracy of the data collected by the laboratory is first assessed using same samples, reagents and standards that have been previously used. This helps to identify if any lab error or instrumental error or analyst error caused the OOS result. Common causes of error include faulty dilutions, incorrect calculations, equipment malfunction and error in analytical method adopted.

If none of these are identified as the cause, the investigation moves to the second phase which is a full-scale OOS investigation.

Phase II: Full-scale OOS Investigation

In this phase, a multi-department investigation committee is formed with representatives from QC, QA, Production, Stores and Engineering. Tthe production process is reviewed and if necessary, additional laboratory analysis is performed. Sampling procedures, production processes, storage conditions, facility environment are all reviewed to identify the cause of the OOS result. If the cause is successfully identified, the investigation is terminated, and the affected product must be rejected. Other batches of products already distributed, but which may have been affected by the OOS, must also be investigated.

In some cases, the OOS result investigation may be inconclusive – that is, either the OOS result is not confirmed or the cause of the OOS result is not detected. In such situations, the QC unit may decide to release the batch if the following conditions all exist:

- Subsequent re-test results lie within specifications, and
- No laboratory error is identified, and
- No process aberrations have been revealed by the review, and
- Results from the batch's in-process tests, dissolution, content uniformity and other important tests mach the passing re-test results
- The process is found to be robust, and other batches have not been affected.

All findings in all stages of the investigation must be clearly documented and stored.

Documentation of OOS result investigation:

Information to be documented for every OOS result investigation:

- Reason for investigation.
- Details of the OOS result.
- Phase I Laboratory investigation details and findings.
- Summary of Phase II analysis performed.
- Root cause identified as actual/probable cause of the OOS result.
- Description of corrective actions taken following the OOS result.
- Result from document review of previous batches to check if similar problem has occurred before.

Flow of events in case of OOS result:

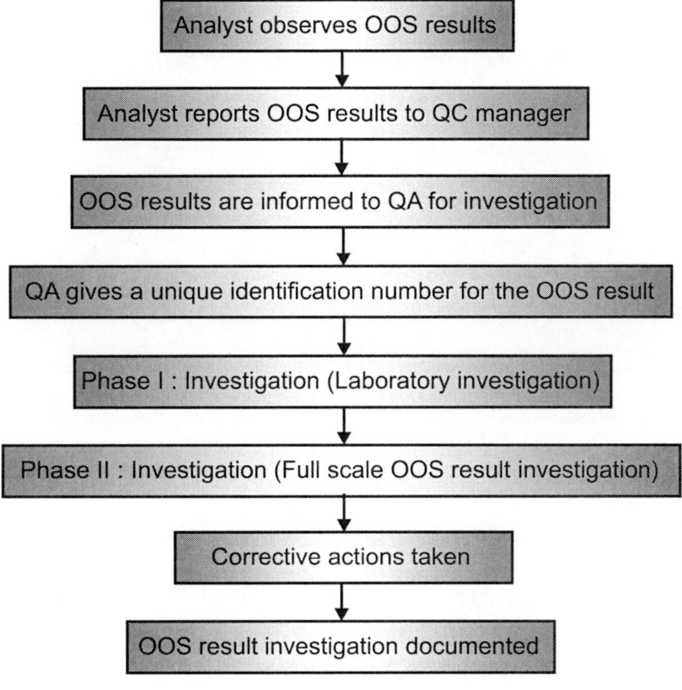

Fig. 10.1

10.11 DRUG PACKAGING

Merely producing a good quality drug product is not enough; it must be packed in a system that ensures the drug retains its activity, efficacy and safety. The packaging used must not have an adverse impact on the drug product; at the same time, it is also important to ensure that the product does not cause damage of the packaging.

10.12 FUNCTIONS OF PACKAGING

The packing material used to deliver a product has several functions:

1. Containment of product is the basic function. The packaging must be effective enough to hold the product without leaking and not cause diffusion of the product.
2. Packaging gives protection against external environmental conditions that may affect the strength, identity, purity and quality of the product.
3. It helps to identify the product by name, and provides all necessary information about the product.
4. Packaging permits the easy use or administration of the drug product.

10.13 CLASSIFICATION OF PHARMACEUTICAL PACKAGING

Packaging materials may be classified into three categories:

1. Primary packaging which first covers the product and holds it – the parts that come into direct contact with the product. Examples – bottle, ampoule, ointment tube etc.
2. Secondary packaging which surrounds the primary packaging. Examples – box, carton, injection tray etc.
3. Tertiary packaging that is used for transportation in bulk. Examples – barrel, crate etc.

Materials commonly used in packaging

Material type	Used for
Glass	Bottles, ampoules, vials, syringes, cartridges
Plastic	Bottles, tubes, closures, bags
Metal	Needles, collapsible tubes, cans, foils, pressurized containers
Rubber	Closures
Cardboard	Boxes
Paper	Labels, information leaflets

10.14 QUALITY CONTROL OF PACKAGING MATERIALS

The physical and chemical characteristics of packaging material are crucial in determining if it will be able to provide adequate containment and protection to the drug product. Packaging material must be designed keeping in mind the nature of the drug product. QC testing of packaging materials is to be done when the materials are received from the vendor; during the packing process and at the end of packing too, samples are drawn to test the completeness and integrity of the final pack.

10.15 PARAMETERS TESTED

Packaging materials are tested for their appearance, dimensions, compatibility, chemical composition and customer usability. Tests are performed to check suitability of:

(a) Material of primary packaging – chemical tests, mechanical tests and environmental tests.

(b) Final pack in secondary packaging – mechanical tests and environmental tests.

Some Important Chemical Tests:

Tests for glass containers:

- Water attack test
- Hydrolytic resistance test
- Powdered glass test
- Light transmission test
- Arsenic test
- Internal bursting pressure test
- Thermal shock test
- Annealing test
- Vertical load test
- Autoclaving

Ampoule sealing tests:

- Appearance
- Quality of seal
- Sealed ampoule length
- Head space oxygen

Plastic containers testing:

- Physicochemical tests on aqueous extracts
- Heavy metals test
- Non-volatile residue
- Biological in-vivo test
- Haemolytic effect of aqueous extracts
- Acute systemic toxicity

Rubber closure testing:

- Self sealability test
- Fragmentation test

Collapsible tubes testing:

- Leakage test
- Lacquer compatibility test
- Lacquer curing test

Strip and blister packs testing:

- Leakage test

Paper and board tests:

- Paper and board density
- Moisture content
- Air permeability
- Folding endurance
- Grammage
- Tear strength
- Tensile strength
- Burst strength
- Puncture resistance
- Cobb test for water absorbance
- Creasability
- Stiffness
- Rub resistance
- Ink absorbency
- Brightness
- Roughness/smoothness

Tests on cartons:

- Compression
- Coefficient of friction
- Carton opening force
- Crease stiffness
- Joint shear strength

Types of glass containers used in pharmaceutical industry

Type of glass	Composition	Suitable for
Type I	Borosilicate	All injectables (acid, neutral or alkaline pH)
Type II	Soda lime silica with treated inner surface to increase hydrolytic resistance	Acidic and neutral parenterals
Type III	Soda lime silica	Non-aqueous injectables in powder form, non-parenterals
Type IV	General purpose soda lime	Topical and oral dosage forms

10.16 TESTS ON CONTAINERS AS PER INDIAN PHARMACOPOEIA

10.16.1 Tests on Glass Containers

10.16.1.1 Hydrolytic Resistance Test

The tests to be done for defining the type of glass are given in Table 10.1.

Table 10.1

Type of container	Test to be done
Type I and type II glass containers to distinguish from Type III glass containers.	Test 1 (surface test).
Type I and type II glass containers where it is necessary to determine whether the high hydrolytic resistance is due to the chemical composition or the surface treatment.	Test 1 and 2.

Test 1

Carry out the determination on the unused containers. The number of containers to be examined and the volumes of test solution to be used are given in Table 10.2.

Table 10.2

Nominal capacity of container (ml)	Number of containers to be used	Volume of test solution to be used for titration (ml)
Upto 3	At least 20	25
5 or less	At least 10	50
6 - 30	At least 5	50
More than 30	At least 3	100

Remove any debris or dust from the containers. Rinse each container at least twice with water at room temperature. Just before the test, rinse each container with freshly prepared distilled water and allow to drain. Complete the cleaning procedure from the first rinsing in not less than 20 minutes and not more than 25 minutes. Fill the containers to the brim with freshly prepared distilled water, empty them and determine the average overflow volume.

Heat closed ampoules on a water bath or in an air oven at about 50°C. Fill the ampoules with freshly prepared distilled water to the maximum volume compatible with sealing them by fusion of the glass, and seal them. Fill bottles or vials to 90% of their calculated overflow volume and cover them with borosilicate glass dishes or aluminium foil previously rinsed with freshly prepared distilled water. Place the containers in an autoclave containing water so that they remain clear of the water. Close the autoclave, displace the air by the passage of steam for 10 minutes, raise the temperature from 100 to 121°C over 20 minutes, maintain a temperature of 121°C for 60 minutes and reduce the temperature from 121°C to 100°C over 40 minutes, venting to prevent vacuum. Remove the containers from the autoclave and cool them in a bath of running tap water. Carry out the following titration within 1 hour of removing the containers from the autoclave. Combine the liquids from the containers under examination, measure the volume of test solution specified in Table 10.2 into a conical flask and add 0.15 ml of methyl red solution for each 50 ml of liquid. Titrate with 0.01 M hydrochloric acid taking as the end point the colour obtained by repeating the operation using the same volume of freshly prepared distilled water. The difference between the preparations represents the volume of 0.01M hydrochloric acid required by the test solution. Calculate the volume of 0.01M hydrochloric acid required for each 100 ml of test solution if necessary. The result is not greater than the value stated in Table 10.3.

Table 10.3

Capacity of container (corresponding to 90% average overflow volume in ml)	Volume of 0.01M hydrochloric acid per 100 ml of test solution	
	Type I or Type II glass (ml)	Type III glass (ml)
Not more than 1	2	20
More than 1 but not more than 2	1.8	17.6
More than 5 but not more than 10	1	10.2
More than 10 but not more than 20	0.80	8.1
More than 20 but not more than 50	0.60	6.1
More than 50 but not more than 100	0.50	4.8
More than 100 but not more than 200	0.40	3.8
More than 200 but not more than 500	0.30	2.9
More than 500	0.20	2.2

Test 2:

Examine the number of containers indicated in Table 10.2. Rinse the containers twice with water and then fill completely with a 4% v/v solution of hydrofluoric acid and allow to stand at room temperature for 10 minutes. Empty the containers and rinse carefully 5 times with water. Carry out the procedure described under hydrolytic resistance. Compare the results with the limiting values given in Table 10.3. For type I glass, the values obtained with the hydrofluoric acid treated containers are closely similar to those stated in the table for type I or type II glass. For type II glass, the values obtained with the hydrofluoric acid treated containers greatly exceed those given in the table for type I or type II glass and are similar to those given for type III glass.

10.16.1.2 Powdered Glass Test

Rinse thoroughly six or more containers with purified water selected randomly and dry them with a current of clean dry air. Crush the containers into fragments about 25 mm in size. Divide about 100g of the coarsely crushed glass into three approximately equal portions and place one portion in a mortar and crush the glass further by striking 3 or 4 blows with a hammer. Empty the mortar contents into sieve no. 20, sieve no. 40 and sieve no. 50. Repeat the operation into two remaining portions of glass. Shake the sieve for short time then remove the glass from the sieve. Repeat this crushing and sieving operation. Empty the receiving pan. Transfer the portion retained on the sieve no. 50 which should weigh in excess of 10 g in a closed container and store in a dessicator until used for the test. Spread the specimen on glazed piece of paper and pass a magnet through it to remove the particles of iron that may introduce during the crushing. Transfer the specimen to a 250 ml conical flask of resistant glass and washed with six 30 ml of acetone. Swirling each for about 30 sec and carefully decanting the acetone. Dry the flask and contents for 20 min at 140°C. Transfer the grains to a weighing bottle and cool in a dessicator. Use the test specimen within 4-8 hrs of drying.

Procedure:

Transfer 10 g of the prepared specimen accurately weighed, to a 250 ml conical flask that has been digested previously with high purified water in a bath at 90°C for at least 24 hrs or 121°C for one hour. Add 50 ml of high purity water to this flask and to one similarly prepared blank.

Cap all flasks with borosilicate glass beaker. Place the container in the autoclave and close it securely, leaving the vent hole open. Heat until steam comes out heavily from the vent cock and continue heating for 10 min. Close the vent cock and adjust the temperature to 111°C. Hold the temperature at 121°C for 30 min. Reduce the heat so that the autoclave cools and comes to atmospheric pressure. Detain the water from the flask into a suitably cleaned vessel and wash the residual powdered glass with 4×15 ml high purity water. Add the decanted water to the main wash. Add 5 g of methyl red solution and titrate immediately with 0.02 N sulphuric acid. If the volume of the titrating solution is expected to be less than 10 ml, use a micro burette. Record the volume of 0.02 N sulphuric acid used to neutralize the extract from 10g of specified specimen of glass, corrected for blank. The volume does not exceed indicated in table for the type of glass concerned.

Test limits for powdered glass test

Type	General description	ml of 0.02 N acid
I	Highly resistant borosilicate glass	1.0
II	Sodalime glass	8.5

10.16.1.3 Arsenic Test

Glass containers for aqueous parenteral preparations should comply with the following test. Carry out the test on ampoules the inner and outer surfaces of which are washed 5 times with freshly distilled water.

Prepare a test solution as described in the test for hydrolytic resistance for an adequate number of containers to produce 50 ml. Pipette 10 ml of the test solution from the combined contents of all the containers into a flask, add 10 ml of nitric acid and evaporate to dryness on a water bath. Dry the residue in an oven at 130°C for 30 minutes. Cool, add to the residue 10 ml of hydrazine molybdate reagent, swirl to dissolve and heat under reflux on a water bath for 20 minutes. Cool to room temperature. Determine the absorbance of the resulting solution at the maximum at about 840 nm using 10 ml of hydrazine molybdate reagent as the blank. The absorbance of the test solution does not exceed the absorbance obtained by repeating the determination using 0.1 ml of arsenic standard solution (10 ppm As) in place of the test solution (0.1 ppm).

10.16.2 Metal Containers for Eye Ointments

Metal collapsible tubes comply with the following tests for metal particles.

Select a sample of 50 tubes from the lot to be tested and clean each tube by vibration and/or blowing. Fill the tubes with suitable molten eye ointment base, close the open end of each tube by a double fold and allow the filled tubes to cool overnight at a temperature of 15°C - 20°C. Assemble a metal bacteriological filter with a 4.25 cm filter paper of suitable porosity supported on suitable perforated plate in place of the standard sintered carbon disc and heat it in a suitable manner to a temperature above the melting range of the base. Remove the caps from the cooled tubes, and apply uniform pressure to the closed end of each tube in turn, in such a manner that the time taken to express as much of the base as possible through each nozzle is not less than 20 seconds. Collect the extruded base from the 50 tubes in the heated filter, applying suction to the stem of the filter in order to draw the molten base through the filter paper. When the entire melted base has been removed, wash the walls of the filter and the filter paper with three successive quantities each of 30 m, of chloroform, allow the filter paper to dry and immediately mount it between glasses for examination.

Examine the filter paper under oblique lighting with the aid of magnifying glass with a graticule of 1 mm squares, 1 of which is subdivided into 0.2 mm squares and note:

The number of all metal particles 1 mm in length and longer.

The number in the range 0.5 mm to less than 1 mm and the number in the range 0.2 mm to less than 0.5 mm.

Carry out two further examinations with the filter paper in two different positions so that the lighting comes from different directions and calculate the average number of metal particles counted in each of the three ranges specified. Give each metal particle detected on the filter paper, a score as follows and add the scores together.

Particle size	Score
Particles 1 mm and above	50
Particles 0.5 mm but less than 1 mm	10
Particles 0.2 mm but less than 0.5 mm	02
Particles less than 0.2 mm	Nil

The lot of tubes passes the test if the total score is less than 100 points. If the total score is more than 150 points, the lot fails the test. If the total score is between 100 and 150 inclusive, the test is repeated on a further sample of 50 tubes and the lot passes the test if the sum of the total scores in the two tests is less than 150 points.

10.16.3 Plastic Containers and Closures

10.16.3.1 For Non-parenteral Preparations

10.16.3.1.1 Leakage Test

Fill 10 containers with water, fit with the intended closures and keep them inverted at room temperature for 24 hours. There are no signs of leakage from any container.

10.16.3.1.2 Collapsibility Test

This test is applicable to containers which are to be squeezed in order to remove the contents. A container, by collapsing inward during use, yields at least 90% of its nominal contents at the required rate of flow at ambient temperature.

10.16.3.2 For Oral Liquids

10.16.3.2.1 Clarity of Aqueous Extract

Select, unlabeled and unmarked and non-laminated portions from suitable containers taken at random, sufficient to yield a total area of sample required, taking into account the surface area of both the sides. Cut these portions into strips, none of which has a total area of more than 20 cm^2. Wash the strips free from extraneous matter by shaking them with at least two separate portions of distilled water for about 30 seconds in each case, then draining off the water thoroughly. Select cut and washed portions of the sample with a total surface area of 1250 cm^2, transfer to a flask, previously cleaned with chromic acid mixture and rinsed with several portions of distilled water and add 250 ml of distilled water. Cover the flask with a beaker and autoclave at 121°C for 30 minutes. Carry out a blank determination using 250 ml of distilled water. Cool and examine the extract. It is colourless and free from turbidity.

10.16.3.2.2 Non-volatile Residue

Evaporate 100 ml of the extract obtained in the test for clarity of aqueous extract to dryness and dry to constant weight at 105°C. The residue weighs not more than 12.5 mg.

10.16.3.2.3 Water Vapour Permeability

Fill 5 containers with nominal volume of water and heat seal the bottles with aluminium foil. Weigh accurately each container and allow to stand for 14 days at humidity of 60 ± 5% and temperature of 20°C and 25°C. Reweigh the containers. Loss in weight in each container is not more than 0.2%

10.16.3.2.4 Leakage Test, Collapsibility Test

Comply with test described under plastic containers for non-parenteral preparations.

10.16.3.3 For Parenteral Preparations

Solution S: Fill a container to its nominal capacity with water and close it. If possible, using the usual means of closure; otherwise close using a sheet of pure aluminium. Heat in an autoclave so that a temperature of 121 ± 2°C is reached within 20 to 30 minutes and maintain at this temperature for 30 minutes. If heating at 121°C leads to deterioration of the container, heat at 100°C for 2 hours. Use solution S within 4 hours of preparation.

Blank: Prepare a blank by heating water in a borosilicate flask closed by a sheet of pure aluminium at the temperature and for the time used for the preparation of solution S.

10.16.3.3.1 Clarity and Colour of solution S. Solution S is clear and colourless.

10.16.3.3.2 Acidity or Alkalinity

To a volume of solution S corresponding to 4% of the nominal capacity of the container, add 0.1 ml of phenolphthalein solution. The solution is colourless. Add 0.4 ml of 0.01 M sodium hydroxide. The solution is pink. Add 0.8 ml of 0.01M hydrochloric acid and 0.1 ml of methyl red solution. The solution is orange-red or red.

10.16.3.3.3 Light Absorption

The light absorption in the range of 230 nm to 360 nm of solution S using a blank prepared as described under solution S is not more than 0.20.

10.16.3.3.4 Reducing Substances

To 20 ml of solution S, add 1 ml of dilute sulphuric acid and 20 ml of 0.02 M potassium permanganate. Boil for 3 minutes. Cool immediately. Add 1 g of potassium iodide and titrate immediately with 0.01M sodium thiosulphate using 0.25 ml of starch solution as indicator. Carry out a titration using 20 ml of the blank prepared under light absorption. The difference between the titration volumes is not more than 1.5 ml.

10.16.3.3.5 Transparency

Fill the container previously used for the preparation of solution S to its nominal capacity with a 1 in 200 dilution of the standard suspension for a container made from polyethylene or polypropylene. For containers of other materials use a 1 in 400 dilution. The cloudiness of the suspension is perceptible when viewed through the container and compared with a similar container filled with water.

Tests on unlabeled, unprinted or non-laminated container material includes test for barium, heavy metals, tin, zinc and residue on ignition to be performed as per Indian Pharmacopoeia.

10.16.3.4 Biological Tests

These tests are designed to determine the biological response of animals to plastics and other polymeric material by the injection or instillation of specific extracts from the material under test. Some of the tests performed include:

10.16.3.4.1 Systemic Injection Test

To measure the irritation and toxicity caused by administration of sample orally, on the skin and by inhalation.

Test animal: Albino Mice Inject each of 5 mice in test group with sample or blank observe the animals immediately, again after 4 hours, and then at 24, 48 and 72 hours. If none of animals shows significant greater biological reactivity than the blank, the sample meets the requirements. If abnormal behavior such as prostration or convulsions occur or if there is a loss of body weight greater than 2g, the sample does not meet the requirements.

10.16.3.4.2 Intracutaneous Test

To measure localized irritation and toxicity when sample comes into contact with live subdermal tissues. Test animal- Rabbit Administer intracutaneous injection of doses of the sample and the blank. Examine the sites of for any tissue reaction like erythema, edema, neuosis at 24, 48, 72 hours after injection. Limit- difference between the scores of sample and blank should be lesser than 1.0.

10.16.3.5 Plastic Containers for Ophthalmic preparations

10.16.3.5.1 They should comply with the following tests tests described under plastic containers for non-parenteral preparations.

- Leakage tests
- Collapsibility tests
- Clarity of aqueous extract
- Non-volatile residue
- Comply with the

10.16.3.5.2 Systemic injection test and intracutaneous tests under plastic containers for parenteral preparations.

10.16.3.5.3 Eye irritation Test

Test animals: Healthy rabbits without visible eye irritation.

Extracting media: Sodium chloride injection or vegetable oil.

Procedure:

Use 3 albino rabbits for each extract to be examined. Gently pull the lower lid away from the eyeball to form a cup and instill about 100 microliter of sterile water for injection. Hold the lid together for about 30 seconds. Instill into the other eye 100 microliter of the sample extract prepared as directed under systemic injection test. Examine the eyes 24, 48 and 72 hours after instillation. The requirements of the test are met if the sample extracts show no significant irritant response during the observation period over that with the blank extract. If the irritation is observed in the control eye treated with sterile water for injection, repeat the test using three additional rabbits.

10.16.4 Rubber Closures for Parenteral Product Containers

Rubber closures are generally used for vials and need to be thoroughly tested because they come into direct contact with the injectable preparations. Due to their complex composition, problems may be found with rubber stoppers such as absorbing of the active ingredient or excipients, and leaching of the rubber ingredients into the drug product. This may affect the safety of the product for its intended use. Therefore, a series of tests are performed to evaluate the quality of rubber closures. These include:

Identification – using IR spectroscopy.

Total ash – using compendial methods.

Other Tests:

Sample preparation (Solution A): Wash the closures in 0.2% w/v of anionic surface active agents for 5 min. Rinse 5 times with distilled water and add 200 ml water and is subjected to autoclave at 119°C to 123°C for 20 to 30 minutes covering with aluminum foil. Cool and separate solution from closure to obtain Solution A.

10.16.4.1 Sterilization Test

When treated closures are subjected to sterilization test at 64°C to 66°C and a pressure of about 0.7 kPa for 24 hours, the closures must not soften or become tacky and there shall be no visual change in the closure.

10.16.4.2 Fragmentation Test

This is applicable to closures intended to be pierced by a hypodermic needle. For closures that are intended to be used for aqueous preparations, place a volume of water corresponding to the nominal volume – 4 ml in each of the 12 clean vials, close the vials with the prepared closures, secure with a cap and allow to stand for 16 hours. For closures that are intended to be used for dry preparations, close 12 clean vials with the prepared closures. Using a lubricated long bevel hypodermic needle with an external diameter of 0.8 mm fitted to a clean syringe, inject 1 ml of water into the vial and remove 1 ml of air; carry out this operation 4 times for each closure, piercing each time at a different site. Use a new needle for each closure and check that the needle is not blunted during the test. Pass the liquid in the vials through a filter with a nominal pore size of 0.5 micrometer. Count the number of fragments visible to the naked eye. The total number of fragments is not more than

10 except in case of butyl rubber closures where the total number of fragments is not more than 15.

10.16.4.3 Self-sealability Test

This is applicable to closures intended to be used with multidose containers. Fill 10 suitable vials with water to the nominal volume, close the vials with the prepared closures and secure with a cap. For each closure, use a new hypodermic needle with an external diameter of 0.8 mm and pierce the closure 10 times, piercing each time at a different site. Immerse the vials upright in a 0.1% w/v solution of methylene blue and reduce the external pressure by 27 kPa for 10 minutes. Restore the atmospheric pressure and leave the vials immersed for 30 minutes. Rinse the outside of the vials. None of the vials contain any trace of coloured solution.

10.16.4.4 pH of Aqueous Extract

20 ml of solution A is mixed with 0.1 ml bromothymol blue and a small amount of 0.01 M sodium hydroxide is added to change the colour from blue to yellow. The volume of sodium hydroxide required is not more than 0.3 ml and if it is done with 0.01 M hydrochloric acid, the volume of acid needed should be not more than 0.8 ml.

10.16.4.5 Reducing Substances

20 ml of solution A is mixed with 1 ml of 1 M sulphuric acid and 20 ml of 0.002 M potassium permanganate and boiled for 3 minutes, and cooled immediately. 1 g of potassium iodide is added and solution is titrated against sodium thiosulphate using starch as an indicator. Blank is done and the difference between titration volumes is not more than 0.7 ml.

10.16.4.6 Residue on Evaporation

50 ml of solution A is evaporated to dryness at 105°C. The residue weight must be not more than 4 mg.

10.17 TESTS FOR PAPER AND BOARDS

10.17.1 Dimensions

The length, breadth and height of the sample material are measured.

10.17.2 Thickness

This is measured using a micrometer; its value depends on grammage and bulk density of test material.

10.17.3 Grammage

A piece measuring 10cm x 10 cm is cut and weight is recorded. Grammage is calculated as:

$$\text{Grammage} = \frac{\text{Weight of sample in grams} \times 1000}{\text{Area of sample in cm}^2}$$

10.17.4 pH of Surface

Chemical residues can cause pH to become acidic. pH is tested by placing a drop of distilled water on top of the test piece and placing the electrode of the pH meter in the drop touching the paper. Reading is measured after 2 minutes.

10.17.5 pH of Extract

1 gram of paper is cut and placed in a 100 ml flask which is fitted with a condenser. 20 ml boiling distilled water is added little by little till the paper is wet. Then 50 ml of distilled water is added, and this is refluxed with occasional shaking at 95°C - 100°C for 1 hour. The mixture is cooled to 40°C to 45°C and the flask is detached from the condenser, shaken and cooled in water bath. The pH of the supernatant is determined using the pH meter.

10.17.6 Alkalinity

5 grams of sample is weighed, cut into pieces and placed in a stoppered flask with 250 ml of 0.02 N hydrochloric acid. After standing for 1 hour, the supernatant is decanted and a measured quantity (V) is titrated against 0.1 N sodium hydroxide with methyl orange indicator. A blank is also performed and alkalinity is calculated as:

$$\text{Percentage alkalinity} = \frac{1250 \ (B - A) \times N}{V \times w}$$

where B = blank titre value, A = sample titre value, N = normality of sodium hydroxide, V = measured quantity used in titration and w = weight of paper taken

10.17.7 Moisture Content

Specimen weight is recorded and it is heated to a constant weight to remove moisture. The final weight is recorded and the difference between the two weights is the moisture content of the paper.

10.17.8 Ash Content

1 gram of specimen is shredded and placed in a weighed crucible. The crucible is heated until contents are completely charred. The crucible is transferred to a muffle furnace at 800° until carbonaceous material is burnt off. Then it is cooled in a dessicator, weighed and experiment is repeated until a constant weight is obtained.

$$\% \text{ ash} = \frac{100 \ (C - D)}{D}$$

where C = initial weight of crucible, D = final weight of crucible.

10.17.9 Cobb Test

This test is a measurement of the mass of water absorbed by 1 cm^2 of test piece in a specified time when submerged under 1 cm of water. The result is quoted in grams/meter^2

10.17.10 Other Tests for Paper/Board/Cartons

Some of the other important tests for paper/board/cartons are as described below:

Folding endurance	Test piece is folded back and forth till it ruptures.
Tear strength	Mean force required to continue tearing of initial cut in a single sheet of paper.
Tensile strength	Maximum tensile force per unit width a paper is capable of withstanding before it breaks.
Burst strength	The maximum uniformly distributed pressure, applied at a right angle to the surface that a test piece of paper can withstand under conditions of test.
Puncture resistance	Energy needed to make initial puncture.
Rub resistance	How resistant printed material is to withstand rubbing.
Compression	Strength of erected package is assessed.
Crease stiffness	Carton board piece is folded through 90° and its ability to recover original position when bending force is removed is tested.
Carton opening force	Test to measure side seam glued cartons to check resistance to erection.
Joint shear strength	Test for strength of adhesive that glues the lap seam on the side of the carton.
Roughness and smoothness	To check surface for ease of printability.

REVIEW QUESTIONS

1. Define QC and explain its role in the pharmaceutical industry.
2. Explain the organization and functions of the QC unit.
3. Describe the sampling and testing procedures followed by QC.
4. Define the term OOS result. How is investigation of such results performed?

5. Classify packing materials used in the pharmaceutical industry.

6. Name and explain the different types of glass used for packaging pharmaceutical products.

7. Explain tests performed on glass containers for parenteral use.

8. Describe the tests to be performed on rubber closures.

9. Discuss the tests for plastic containers for ophthalmic preparations.

10. List and discuss the tests for paper and board used to make cartons.

✍ ✍ ✍

GOOD LABORATORY PRACTICES FOR NON-CLINICAL LABORATORIES

Objectives:

Upon completion of this section, the student should be able to

- Define the term 'Good Laboratory Practices' and explain its scope.
- Describe the organization and management systems in a non-clinical testing facility.
- Explain requirements of a testing facility with respect to personnel, premises, facilities and utilities.
- Outline the precautions to be taken in animal and material handling in a non-clinical test facility.
- Describe the documentation to be maintained by a testing facility.
- Outline the reasons for disqualification of a testing facility and disqualification procedures.

Introduction

In 1976, the United States Food and Drug Adminsitration (USFDA) received information from a whistleblower about some problems in data submitted by a company called Syntex. Erroneously, an FDA official picked up a file on a contract laboratory called IBT (Industrial Bio-Test Laboratories) which was under contract to Syntex.

On reviewing the data submitted by IBT, serious defects in the study were found, and the FDA performed an inspection of the IBT facility where even more shocking critical deficiencies in scientific procedures were unearthed. It was found that data was being fabricated, adverse health effect results were being removed from reports, dead study animals were being replaced with healthy ones, histopathology data was being fudged and report conclusions were being modified to make the drug appear favourable.

A little later, similar malpractices were found in the long-term toxicology studies being conducted in laboratories of the company called G.D. Searle and Company.

Suspecting that similar situations existed in most research facilities throughout the pharmaceutical sector, the FDA decided to institute a monitoring program to ensure sound and scientific laboratory practices were followed.

In august 1976, draft proposal for Good Laboratory Practice (GLP) regulations was published in the Federal Register on 19th November 1976. These regulations laid down a uniform approach to ensure the integrity of data produced during non-clinical laboratory studies. By creating a system of Quality Assurance (QA) unit in testing laboratories, it was sought to ensure that the facility complied with regulatory requirements. On 4th September, 1987, the Good Laboratory Practice Regulations, The Final Rule, were published.

11.1 DEFINITION OF GLP

FDA defines GLP as, "A set of principles intended to assure the quality and integrity of non-clinical laboratory studies that are intended to support research or marketing permits for products regulated by government agencies."

The term non-clinical laboratory study refers to the *in-vitro* or *in-vivo* experiments where item being tested is studied in systems under laboratory conditions to evaluate how safe it will be.

Thus, GLP ensures that testing facilities comply with the minimum requirements the FDA expects with respect to the planning, conducting and reporting of safety studies related to non-clinical testing. By providing a framework for a well-controlled study, GLP assure an overall accountability.

11.2 SCOPE OF GLP

The term GLP applies to the non-clinical testing required for approval of new drug products for human and animal use. Its scope also extends to cover non-pharmaceutical compounds like food additives, colour additives, food packaging, food contamination limits, biological products, electronic products and medical devices.

If a firm hires the services of a contract laboratory or a consultant laboratory service for the testing, that laboratory must also abide by GLP.

The testing laboratory must permit an inspection of their facility and records of the studies being conducted by a duly authorized employee of the FDA.

GLP **does not cover** human clinical studies, discovery-related toxicology studies, non-clinical pharmacology studies to study efficacy and drug action and bioanalysis of samples drawn from clinical trials.

11.3 PERSONNEL

Persons involved in conducting or supervising the study in the non-clinical laboratory must have the necessary education, training and experience to ensure that they can perform their functions adequately. The details of these must be maintained in current condition.

Sufficient personnel must be employed for conducting the study as per the protocol. They must take all due precautions with respect to personal health and sanitation to prevent contaminating the test systems and articles. Clothing of personnel must be apt for their duty; it must be changed as required to avoid chemical, microbiological or radiological contamination during testing.

Any person with an illness that could adversely affect the integrity and quality of the study must be excluded from it until full recovery.

11.4 ORGANIZATION AND MANAGEMENT OF TEST FACILITY

11.4.1 Study Director

Before start of a study, the management of the facility should appoint a study director. This person should be either a scientist or a professional who has the necessary education, training and experience to manage the technical aspects of the study and also interpret, analyze, document and report the study results.

11.4.2 Systems

Test protocol should be prepared and approved by authorized person. All data collected during experiments must be recorded accurately and verified, including unanticipated responses. If any situation occurs that may affect the quality and integrity of the study, it must be noted, and corrective action must be taken and documented. All GLP regulations that apply to the study must be followed and testing must be carried out as laid out in the protocol. At the close of the study, all data, documents, samples and final reports must be archived safely.

11.4.3 Management

The management of test facility must make sure that all materials, facilities, resources, equipment and personnel required for testing are available. It must also assure that tests for identity, purity, strength, stability and uniformity, as applicable, have been performed adequately. Personnel must understand the functions they are to perform. Deviations if observed must be reported by QA unit directly to the study director; corrective actions must be taken and documented.

11.4.4 QA Unit

A quality assurance unit must be set up in a manner as to be independent of the persons involved with the study. There must be written procedures, and details of responsibilities and records to be maintained by this unit.

This unit must monitor that equipment, facilities, personnel, practices, methods, records and controls match the GLP regulations. It is this unit's responsibility to have all information – a master schedule sheet, protocols etc – of the studies performed by the lab. The QA unit must inspect the study regularly to verify the study integrity, and these inspections must be documented with signatures. Any problems that can compromise the integrity of the study must be reported to the study director and the management at once.

QA unit must provide written status reports of the study at regular intervals to the study director. Any problems and the corrective actions taken must be clearly indicated. The unit must also ensure that no deviations from the standard operating procedures (SOPs) or protocol occur without duly documented authorization.

It is also the responsibility of QA unit to review the study report at the end and check that it gives an accurate description of the methods, and that the results being reported match the findings as per the raw data generated in the study.

All QA documents must be made available for inspection by the authorized FDA representative.

11.5 FACILITIES

The testing facility must be of a suitable size and constructed to allow proper conduct of the study, without any adverse effect on the study.

11.5.1 Animal Care Facilities

There must be enough animal areas or rooms to allow separation of different species/test systems. Each project must be run in isolation. Housing and quarantine requirements of the animals must be sufficiently met. There must be entirely separate rooms and areas to carry out studies on materials that are biohazardous (such as aerosols, infectious agents, volatile substances and radioactive materials). Separate areas must be kept for isolation of animals who are carriers of disease or that have been diagnosed with any disease. Proper arrangements must be made to dispose animal waste without causing odor, environmental contamination, vermin infestation or disease hazards.

11.5.2 Animal Supply Facilities

Space must be provided for storage of animal supplies such as bedding, feed, supplies and equipment. These areas must be kept separate from the test system housing areas, and kept free of contamination or infestation. Perishable supplies must be duly protected.

11.5.3 Test and Control Handling Facilities

Separate areas must exist for receiving and storing control and test articles, and test and control article mixtures, to prevent any contamination or mixup. These storage areas must be designed to prevent any change in the purity, strength, identity and stability of the articles and mixtures.

11.5.4 Laboratory Operation Areas

There must be separate space for the laboratory where the study is to be performed including routine as well as specialized procedures.

11.5.5 Specimen and Data Storage Facilities

There must be enough space to archive specimens and data. Access to this area shall be restricted to only authorized personnel.

11.6 EQUIPMENT

11.6.1 Design and Location

All equipment used to generate, measure or assess data and to control the facility environment must be of a design and capacity sufficient to perform its expected function. The equipment must be located in a manner suitable for operation, cleaning, maintenance and inspection.

11.6.2 Calibration and Maintenance

All equipment in the laboratory must be cleaned, inspected and maintained as per written procedures. Any equipment that generates, measures or assesses data must be regularly calibrated or standardized as required. There must be written SOPs for equipment operation, cleaning, inspection, maintenance and testing/calibration/standardization. The SOPs must also specify the personnel to carry out each operation, and include information of remedial action to be performed if there is equipment malfunction or failure.

All inspections, testing/calibration/standardization procedures and maintenance actions must be recorded. Any non-routine repair work done after malfunction or failure of the equipment must also be documented with details of nature of defect and the remedial action taken.

11.7 TESTING FACILITIES OPERATION

11.7.1 Standard Operating Procedures (SOPs)

Written SOPs and laboratory manuals must be present describing the study methods to be adopted to ensure data quality and integrity. The study director must authorize any deviations from the SOPs and the same must be documented. The manuals and SOPs must be immediately available in the area where the particular task is being performed. Data regarding all versions of SOPs must be maintained including details of revision dates.

Minimum required SOPs in a non-clinical laboratory:

- Preparation of animal room.
- Animal care.
- Test and control articles receiving, identification, handling, storage, mixing and sampling methods.
- Laboratory tests.
- Test system observations.
- Handling of animals found dead in the course of the study.
- Necropsy/post-mortem examination of such animals.
- Collecting and identifying specimens.
- Histopathology study.
- Storage, handling and retrieval of data.
- Calibration and maintenance of equipment.
- Placement and identification of animals and their transfer.

11.7.2 Solutions and Reagents

All solutions and reagents kept and used in the lab must be labeled to show the identity, concentration, expiry date and storage requirements. Outdated substances must not be used.

11.7.3 Animal Care

Care, handling, feeding and housing of animals must be done in keeping with written procedures. When animals are newly received at the laboratory, they must be isolated until their health status is evaluated as per standard veterinary medical practice. Only animals without any disease or condition that may interfere with the conduct or purpose of the study must be used when the study begins. If a disease is contracted by the animals during the study, such animals must be isolated if required. They may be treated for the disease but the treatment should not interfere with the study. Details of all such diagnoses, treatment authorization, its description and the treatment dates must be documented and archived.

Warm-blooded animals being used in the study long-term, or those used in studies where they must be moved in and out of the cages, must be sufficiently identified. Each animal housing unit must bear details of all the animals housed in it. Separate housing must be provided for animals belonging to different species if necessary. Animals of same species must not be kept together if they are being used in different studies as there could be a mix-up that affects the study outcomes. If common housing is unavoidable, care must be taken to allow separation by space and identification.

Cages, equipment, racks must be cleaned and sanitized regularly. The water and feed supplied to the animals must be tested at regular intervals to rule out their contamination. Details of such testing must be documented as raw data. Bedding used in the cages must not interfere with the study; it should be changed often enough to ensure animals are clean and dry. Pest control materials used must be such as to not interfere with the study. Use of such materials must be documented.

11.7.4 Characterization of Test and Control Articles

For every batch of control and test articles, their purity, strength, identity and composition must be determined and documented. Their synthesis method must be documented by either the study sponsor or the testing laboratory. Stability of these articles must be evaluated either before the study begins or along with the study, as per written SOPs.

The containers in which test and control articles are stored must be labeled with appropriate information such as name, code number, batch number, storage conditions and expiry date. Containers must not be changed until the end of the study. When the study duration is longer than 4 weeks, reserve samples must be drawn and retained from each batch of the control and test articles.

11.7.5 Handling of Control and Test Articles

Test and control articles must be handled in a way that they are stored, identified and distributed in a way that avoids contamination or deterioration, and their receiving and distribution (with quantities) is to be documented.

11.7.6 Article-carrier Mixtures

When control or test article is mixed with a carrier, there must be tests performed to ensure mixture uniformity, concentration and stability of the articles in the mixture. Stability may be assessed either before the study commences, or during course of the study according to written SOPs. The expiry date of the mixture must be indicated.

11.8 PROTOCOL FOR AND CONDUCT OF NON-CLINICAL LABORATORY STUDY

11.8.1 Protocol

Written and approved protocols must exist for each study, and they must indicate the purpose of the study and methods to be adopted in conducting the study. The following information must form a part of the protocol:

- Title and purpose statement for the study.

- Test and control articles identified by name, code number or chemical abstract number.
- Study sponsor name, and testing facility name and address.
- Test system being used – number, sex, age, body weight range, species, strain, substrain and supplier details.
- Procedure to identify test system.
- Experimental design description, methods used for bias control.
- Description of items to be used in study – diet of animals, solvents or emulsifiers, and limit values for contaminants likely to be found in these that may interfere with study
- Dosage levels (in mg/kg body weight) of control and test articles; the frequency and method of administration.
- Tests, measurements, analyses to be performed and their frequency.
- Information regarding the statistical methods that will be used in the study.
- Date when study protocol was approved by sponsor, and signature with date by study director.
- Any changes/revisions in an approved protocol must be documented along with the reason; it must be signed and dated by the study director and this document must be kept along with the protocol.

11.8.2 Conduct of the Study

The non-clinical laboratory study must be conducted according to the protocol. All specimens must be labeled with details of study, test system, nature and date of collection. If a specimen is to be examined histopathologically by a pathologist, the gross findings from post-mortem examination must be also available.

Data generated during the course of a study (except automatically collected data) must be recorded at once, directly, and in legible ink. Dates and initials of the person making the entry should be affixed. If any change is to be made, it shall be done in a manner to not deface the original entry. The reason for the change must be documented, and dated and signed. In case of automated data collection systems, the person responsible for data input must be identified. Any changes in data must follow the same procedure as for other means of data collection.

11.9 RECORDS AND REPORTS

11.9.1 Reporting Study Results

Final report must be prepared for each study, containing the following information:
- Name of the facility, address, and dates of study commencement and completion.
- Details of purpose and procedure as per approved protocol, and any changes in protocol.
- Statistical data analysis methods.
- Test and control articles – names, code numbers, purity, strength, composition etc.
- Stability parameters of control and test articles under study conditions.

- Methods used in the study.
- Test system description – details of animal numbers, sex, species, strain and substrain, body weight range, age, identification procedure.
- Details of dose, dosage regimen, duration, route of administration.
- All circumstances that may have had an effect on the data quality or integrity.
- Names of study director, other scientists or professionals, and supervisory personnel who participated in the study.
- Details of calculations and other procedures performed with the data, data analysis and summary, and conclusions inferred from the analysis.
- Dated and signed reports of each scientist/professional who was part of the study.
- Locations of storage of raw data, specimens and final report.
- Prepared statement signed by QA unit.

The study's final report must have the date and signature of study director. Any corrections in the final report must be reported separately as an amendment, and the reasons for correction must be specified, along with date and signature by the person responsible for the correction.

11.9.2 Data and Records Storage and Retrieval

All documents, protocols, raw data, specimens and final reports generated during the study must be retained except wet specimens of urine, blood, feces and biological fluids and the ones from mutagenicity tests. These reports must be stored in an orderly manner to allow easy retrieval when required, with adequate precautions against deterioration of the documents or specimens. Such storage may be done off-premises and details of where it has been stored must be retained in the laboratory.

11.9.3 Retaining Records

Records must be retained for whichever of the following is the shortest duration:
- At least 2 years after the date when application for research or marketing permit (for which the study was conducted) is approved by FDA.
- At least 5 years after the date when results of the study were submitted to FDA to support an application for research or marketing permit.
- At least 2 years after date of study completion or discontinuation or termination, in cases where the study results are not used to support an application for research or marketing permit.
- Wet specimens (except from mutagenicity tests) and wet specimens of urine, blood, biological fluids and feces, and other samples that are fragile and deteriorate on storage must be kept only until their quality allows evaluation.
- Protocol copies, master schedule sheet and QA inspection reports must be stored by the QA unit so as to be easily accessible.
- Job descriptions, summaries of employee training and experience must be retained with other employment records for duration as mentioned in first two points.

- Reports of equipment calibration, inspection and maintenance must be retained.
- Records must be kept either in original form or true copies as photocopies, microfiche, microfilm etc.

In the event that the facility conducting the study goes out of business, all the documentation, raw data and other records must be transferred to the study sponsor for storage, and the FDA must be given written notice of this.

11.10 DISQUALIFICATION OF TESTING FACILITIES

11.10.1 Purpose

Disqualification may serve the following purposes:

1. To exclude from being considered the completed studies that were performed by a facility that has failed to comply with GLP regulations until it can be proved that such non-compliances did not occur during a particular study or that the non-compliances did not affect the acceptability of data generated during that study.

2. To exclude from being considered, all the studies that have been completed following disqualification until the facility undertakes to conduct studies according to GLP regulations.

If a testing facility is disqualified, the sponsor of the study that was performed (and disqualified) cannot use that as an excuse to not submit the study in their application for research or marketing permit. They must get the study repeated and submit with the application.

11.10.2 Disqualification Grounds

Reasons why a testing facility may be disqualified include:

- Failure to comply with one or more of the GLP regulations.
- The non-compliance has created an adverse effect on the validity of the study.
- Previous incidents of warnings or individual study rejections have not helped to achieve compliance with GLP guidelines.

When the FDA has relevant information to justify a test facility disqualification, the Commissioner issues a written notice to the concerned facility proposing the disqualification. A regulatory hearing will then be conducted as per legal guidelines.

11.10.3 Final Disqualification Order

After the regulatory hearing, or after time permitted for a contest by the facility passes without such action, the Commissioner of FDA evaluates the records of the proceedings and issues the final order to disqualify the facility, with the reason for the disqualification. A copy of this order must be sent to the testing facility.

11.10.4 Actions Following Disqualification

After disqualification of a testing facility, scrutiny is done of every application for research or marketing permit that contains data from a study conducted by the disqualified testing facility. It is determined if that study is acceptable or not. If the study is considered unacceptable, the onus lies on the study sponsor to prove that the study was unaffected by the non-compliances that led to the disqualification. This may include validating the data by a repeat study.

Any study done by a disqualified testing facility will be invalid for the purpose of application for a research or marketing permit, unless the facility has been reinstated after due procedure.

11.10.5 Public Disclosure of Disqualification

After a testing facility has been disqualified by the final order, the FDA Commissioner notifies all interested persons at his discretion if he believes the disclosure is in public interest, or that it will promote compliance with GLP. If public notice is given, it must include a copy of final disqualification order along with the statement that the FDA will not consider any studies done by the said facility in support of any application for research or marketing permit.

11.10.6 Termination or Suspension of Testing Facility by Sponsor

If a sponsor suspends or terminates a laboratory from further participation in the study, it must notify the FDA in writing within 15 working days, along with the reasons for such action.

11.10.7 Reinstatement of a Disqualified Testing Facility

The disqualified testing facility may apply to the FDA Commissioner assuring that it will comply with GLP regulations in the future, along with details of the corrective actions that have been taken or are intended to be taken, and the reasons why it believes it must be reinstated. On examining this submission, and following an inspection, if the Commissioner determines that GLP regulations are being followed, he may reinstate the testing facility as a source for the study. The testing facility must be notified and any other involved persons, such as the sponsor, and information about the reinstatement is publicly disclosed.

Before a new drug is introduced into the market, it has to undergo certain *in-vitro* and *in-vivo* experiments in a non-clinical setting. This is usually achieved through a study that involves testing of the drug on animal specimens, or on microbiological or biological test systems. In order for the results of such studies to be valid and authentic, it is vital that the study must have been conducted under conditions that ensure data validity and integrity. GLP guidelines provide information regarding these conditions to be maintained by testing facilities and complying with these is the key to a successful application for a new drug.

REVIEW QUESTIONS

1. Define GLP and discuss its scope.
2. Explain the personnel responsibilities in a non-clinical testing facility.
3. Discuss the important facilities to be provided in testing units where animal testing is performed.
4. Write a note on GLP requirements for documentation in a non-clinical testing laboratory.
5. Describe the grounds on which a testing facility may be disqualified.
6. Explain the steps of a testing facility disqualification by regulatory authorities

Chapter ... **12**

COMPLAINT, RECALLS AND WASTE DISPOSAL

Objectives:

Upon completion of this section, the student should be able to

- Define and classify pharmaceutical market complaints
- Outline the steps involved in handling product complaints
- List the stages in complaint investigation
- Explain the corrective actions taken after investigation of complaints
- Define drug recalls and classify them as per regulatory guidelines
- Cite examples of major drug recalls in history
- Explain the procedure of handling returned goods
- Classify the types of waste produced in a pharmaceutical manufacturing unit
- Explain the waste disposal methods to be used for medicines

Introduction

Despite all precautions taken by a manufacturer, there is always the likelihood that some problem is present in a given drug product. At such times, customers are likely to find fault with either the content or the packaging of the product, and this dissatisfaction is conveyed in the form of a complaint.

It is important that these complaints be investigated, and corrective actions be taken to deal with the complaints as well as any underlying problems responsible for the conditions that lead to the complaint. All pharmaceutical manufacturers are required to have a complaint handling system to address such issues.

There must be written procedures that describe how to handle all oral and written complaints about a drug product. These procedures must lay down the actions to be taken in the event of receiving a complaint.

12.1 STEPS IN COMPLAINT HANDLING

The process of handling complaints may be studied under the following headings:

1. Receiving the complaint
2. Technical examination and investigation of the complaint
3. Corrective measures and giving feedback to complainant
4. Trend analysis

12.1.1 Receiving the Complaint

Companies must provide open channels through which customers can raise their complaints. For example, P.O. box numbers or email ids, or toll-free numbers for complaint filing must be publicized. The company must appoint a person who will be responsible for receiving the complaint, and documenting it as per company requirements.

12.1.2 Technical Examination and Investigation of the Complaint

Once the complaint has been received, a complaint investigation form should be prepared with the following information.

- Name and contact details of the complainant,
- Details of the drug product on which complaint has been raised – product name, manufacturing batch number/lot number, manufacturing and expiry dates, quantity of product where problem is seen, and
- Details of the nature of the complaint – what exactly is wrong and has been complained about.

Product complaint data sheet details:

- Serial number of complaint.
- Complaint details.
- Name and address of complainant.
- Date of receiving complaint.
- Name of person who received the complaint.
- Details of product involved – name, strength, batch number.
- Size of sample obtained from person raising complaint.
- Complaint evaluation report.
- Name and signature of investigators with date.
- Action taken report.
- Copy of written response sent to complainant.

Complaints may be classified as:

(a) Product quality complaints (non-therapeutic) – to be investigated within 5 days.

(b) Packaging complaints (packing error/shortage) – to be investigated within 10 days.

(c) Medical complaints (therapeutic) – to be investigated within 3 days.

This information is sent to the Quality Assurance (QA) department to start investigation. A QA Officer is appointed as Complaint Officer to oversee the next stages. Two phases of investigation will follow: first, a document-based investigation and next, a laboratory analysis.

12.1.3 Document-Based Investigation

This involves review of

(a) Complaint files to see how many previous complaints of a similar nature have occurred, and how the complaints were handled.

(b) Batch manufacturing and packaging records to check for any incidents of non-conformance during that particular batch's processing.

12.1.4 Laboratory Analysis

This phase involves an analysis by the Quality Control (QC) laboratory. The samples received with the complaint as well as the samples that have been retained by the manufacturer must be tested and the results must be documented.

The Complaint Officer compares results of the laboratory analysis and the document-based investigation and prepares a report that may result in on one of three conclusions:

1. **Confirmed complaint:** When out-of-specifications (OOS) results are seen in both complaint and retained samples or in only complaint samples. For example, if both samples of tablets showed discolouration; or one tablet is missing from blister pack in complaint sample but not in retained sample.

2. **Non-confirmed complaint:** When both complaint and retained samples test results comply with specifications or if only complaint sample shows OOS results. For example, tablets in complaint sample are discoloured but this is not seen in retained samples. This could be attributed to improper storage of the drug at point of sale.

3. **Counterfeit/tamper suspicion:** When retained sample meets specifications but complaint sample results are OOS, with no possible reason to explain the deviation. For example, if packing material in complaint sample is totally different from that of retained sample, it could indicate counterfeit drug. Or if colour of complaint sample drug is totally different from retained sample drug, it may indicate tampering.

The Complaint Officer must also investigate if the complaint involves any unexpected or serious adverse drug reaction.

After completion of investigation, generally within 30 days of receiving the complaint, the report is prepared and signed by Complaint Officer and QA Manager.

The complaint file must be maintained for at least one year following expiry date of the concerned product batch.

12.1.5 Corrective Measures and Giving Feedback to Complainant

In case of confirmed complaints, the company must implement corrective actions depending on the severity of the problem. In simple cases, it may be sufficient to impart training of employees; in more complex situations, it may call for launching a Corrective

Action and Preventive Action (CAPA) by putting together a team of representatives from Production, QC, QA and higher management areas.

In case of non-confirmed complaints that may have originated from improper handling of product, the company must send a written response to the complainant, including information on correct method of handling the product. The customer may also be sent a free replacement product along with the response letter.

In case of complaints about serious therapeutic problems or adverse drug reactions in a significant number, the company may decide to opt for a product recall if they foresee a considerable risk in continued sale of the drug.

12.1.6 Trend Analysis

All complaints received must be analyzed and a trend analysis must be performed, to collect relevant information. Some of the areas to be investigated include – how many complaints were received? How many were confirmed, non-confirmed and counterfeit/tamper suspicions?

The complaint file along with the trend analysis reports must be kept available for perusal during cGMP (current Good Manufacturing Practices) audits/inspections.

Complaint files must be maintained till a minimum of one year after expiry of the drug product or till one year after the date of receiving the complaint, whichever is longer. For Over the Counter (OTC) products where there is no expiry date, the files must be maintained for at least 3 years after the product's distribution.

In case of complaints where an investigation was not performed, the file must record this along with the reason for not performing the investigation. This record must also indicate the name of the person who took this decision to not investigate the complaint.

12.2 DRUG RECALLS

Drug recall refers to the action of removing or withdrawing a batch of product from distribution or use, to be returned to the manufacturer. This action is generally done in cases where deficiencies are discovered in the safety, quality or efficacy of drugs. It is important to note that product recall **does not** include the normal removal of products that have passed their expiry period.

The Organization of Pharmaceutical Producers of India (OPPI) defines recall as, "An action taken to resolve a problem with therapeutic goods for which there are established deficiencies in quality, efficacy or safety."

According to the CDSCO (Central Drugs Standard Control Organization), quality defects may include drugs that are not of standard quality, spurious or adulterated drugs. Safety and efficacy defects include serious adverse drug reactions and death. Drugs manufactured despite being prohibited under the provisions of the Drugs and Cosmetics Act, and products manufactured under cancelled or suspended license may also be recalled from the market.

12.2.1 Types of Recall

Product recall may be of two types:

(a) Voluntary recall: This refers to situations when the manufacturer decides on their own initiative to recall products where the safety, efficacy and quality of a batch is in question. For example:

1. Batch does not comply with regulatory requirements during stability study done in the post-marketing phase.
2. An in-house investigation reveals a failure (cross-contamination or mix-up) that may have an adverse effect on the quality of a batch of product that has already been released for distribution.
3. Market complaint investigations show that the entire batch of distributed product is defective.
4. Visual inspection of retained samples show evidence of deterioration that has an impact on product quality.
5. Pharmacovigilance reports indicate a serious safety risk to those taking the medication.

(b) Statutory recall: These are recalls mandated by drug regulatory bodies at Central or State levels for one of the following reasons:

1. The product violates the law – Example, it is not of standard quality.
2. The formulation contains banned drugs.
3. The labeling of the product or promotional material violates the law.
4. Product is found to contravene provisions of Schedule J (it claims to cure a disease/disorder that no drug can claim to do)

Regulatory bodies encourage manufacturers to implement a product recall voluntarily if they discover that any of their products is defective. However, in cases where the regulatory body finds evidence of seriously defective or dangerous products, it may suggest or order a product recall by sending a notice to the concerned company. In case of non-compliance by the company to such an order, legal action may be initiated against the manufacturer.

In cases where the product recall is ordered by the regulatory body, the concerned company may choose to contest the notice. However, it is important to do a complete review of the actual situation and take necessary legal advice before proceeding in this direction.

12.2.2 Recall is Different from Withdrawal

Drug recall is removal from the market due to quality, safety or efficacy issues. Drug withdrawal on the other hand, is a change in the approval status of the drug by the concerned regulatory authorities. If the nature and frequency of adverse drug events is such that the risks of a drug far outweigh its benefits, the regulatory body may decide to withdraw approval for the manufacturing of such a product and the manufacturer is informed to stop producing it.

12.2.3 Reasons for Product Recall

Product recall may have to be carried out if:

- Potentially dangerous/serious product quality issues have come to light through complaints or other means.
- Mandatory regulations have been violated and come to the notice of regulatory agencies, who then order a recall.
- Field monitoring studies/other reports show evidence of tampering with the product.
- New information that comes to light after distribution of a product indicates it is unsafe or ineffective or dangerous.

Most common reasons for drug recalls:

- cGMP violations.
- Microbial contamination in non-sterile products.
- Failing dissolution test requirements.
- Degradation products/impurities.
- Lack of efficacy.
- Labeling errors (declared strength).
- Lack of assurance of sterility.
- Misbranded drug (therapeutic claims that are unapproved in promotional literature).
- Lack of drug stability.
- Incorrect outer packaging (correct label on product, packed in incorrect carton).

12.2.4 Classification of Recall

The CDSCO classifies recalls into three categories:

Class I is the situation in which there is a reasonable probability that the use of, or exposure to, a defective product will cause serious adverse health consequences or death and as well as drugs banned under 26A of Drugs and Cosmetics Act 1940. Recalls under this class must be executed to the level of distributor/wholesaler, retailer and consumer. Public announcements shall be made using print and electronic media. Timeline for recall ranges from within 24 hours up to a maximum of 72 hours – stopping the sale/distribution must be enforced within 24 hours; physical recall must be completed within 72 hours.

Class II is a situation in which the use of, or exposure to, a defective product may cause temporary adverse health consequences or where the probability of serious adverse health consequences is remote. These recalls are implemented at the level of distributor/wholesaler and retailer. Time limit for recall is maximum 10 days.

Class III is a situation in which the use of, or exposure to, a defective product is not likely to cause any adverse health consequences. Here, recall is executed until the wholesaler level, and a time limit of upto 30 days is permitted.

Banned drugs for which license is cancelled or suspended, if found to be in the market, shall have to be recalled, being treated as Class I recall.

12.2.5 Mock Recall

As per CDSCO guidelines, companies must carry out a mock recall for at least one batch of any one of their products after being dispatched. It is best to choose a product where maximum distributors are involved. This helps to evaluate how effective the arrangements are to execute the product recall. Such a mock recall must also be carried out in the event of a change in the marketing/distribution partner. Records of mock recalls must be maintained by the QA department.

USFDA Classification of product recalls

Class I: Situations that involve a threat to life. FDA orders a consumer recall, a 100 % effectiveness check, and requires public announcements to be made about the hazards of the product.

Class II: Situations that is potentially hazardous but not life-threatening. FDA orders recall to retail outlets but a 100% effectiveness check is not mandatory. Depending on reason for the recall, press release may or may not be necessary.

Class III: Situations that do not pose a serious hazard. Recall is restricted to the wholesale outlets. Effectiveness checks are not necessary, no press release is required either.

Product recall guidelines – worldwide

Country	Regulatory body	Guidelines under
USA	Food & Drug Administration (FDA)	21 CFR Parts 7, 107 and 1270.
Australia	Therapeutic Goods Administration (TGA)	Section 65F of the Trade Practices Act 1974.
UK	Medicines and Healthcare products Regulatory Agency (MHRA)	Sections 2(2), 4, 5 and 7 of the European Communities Act 1972 and Directive 2001/95/EC on general product safety.
South Africa	Medicine Control Council	Section 19 (1) of the Medicines and Related Substances Act, Act 101 of 1965 and Regulation 43(1) of the Medicines and Related Substances Control Act, Act 101 of 1965.
India	Central Drugs Standard Control Organization (CDSCO)	Para 27, 28 of Schedule M and conditions of license for defective product recall in Rule 74(j) and Rule 78(i) of the Drugs and Cosmetics Act, 1940 and Rules there under.

Major drug recalls

Product	Company	Category	Year	Reason For Recall
Fenfluramine/ Phentermine	Wyeth-Ayerst	Anti-obesity	1997	Reports of heart valve defects
Phenylpropanolamine (PPA) containing drugs	Many companies	Decongestant		Incidents of haemorrhagic stroke
Baycol	Bayer	Anti-cholesterol	2001	Death linked to rhabdomyolysis
Vioxx	Merck	Anti-inflammatory	2004	Linked to cardiovascular problems
Bextra	Pfizer	Anti-inflammatory	2005	Serious cardiovascular effects and potentially fatal skin conditions
Digitek	Actavis	Heart failure treatment	2008	Double thickness tablets containing double the approved dose
Tylenol	McNeil Consumer Healthcare	Pain reliever	2010	Musty odour of bottles due to preservative sprayed on pallets where bottles were stored.
Excedrin	Novartis	Pain reliever	2012	Suspicion of mix up with other products manufactured at the same premises
Velcade	Takeda Oncology Company	Anti-cancer	2018	Particulate contamination observed after reconstitution
Ranitidine	Several companies	Antacid	2019	Carcinogen nitrosodimethylamine found at levels crossing USFDA limits

12.2.6 Product Recall System

Every company is required to have a product recall system in place to effect a prompt and effective recall in case of serious complaints regarding defective products. As per cGMP guidelines, product recall activities must be coordinated and executed by an authorized person who is independent of the marketing and sales function of the company. The recall approving authority is generally the Head of the Company (President/Proprietor/Managing Director).

Recall strategy details must include information regarding:

1. Authorized person who will initiate the recall.

2. Nature of communication that will be used to initiate recall (telephone, email, letters etc.).

3. Depth of the recall to be instituted (recall from distributor/wholesaler/hospital/ retailer/general public).

4. Manner of receiving, segregating and secure storage of the recalled product.

5. Reconciliation reports to be prepared, at what frequency.

6. Verification of success of recall and report submission to regulatory authorities.

7. Steps to be taken to avoid re-occurrence of the same issue with the product.

8. Dealing with recalled product – reworking or destruction as may be appropriate.

12.3 HANDLING RETURNED GOODS

Once a product recall has been initiated, the process must be monitored to ensure that the recall is completed within the stipulated timeframe. A check must be performed to evaluate the effectiveness of the recall. Following this, an investigation must be carried out to study the reason for the recall and remedial action must be worked out to ensure the defect does not recur.

When stock of recalled drugs is received, it must be placed under quarantine, in a segregated place, with no chance of being mixed up with other products. Entry to this area must be restricted to authorized personnel only. Samples must be drawn and testing performed to identify the root cause of the defects.

Once this has been established, corrective and preventive actions (CAPA) must be drawn up and implemented.

Based on the results of the investigation, the defective product may be re-processed or destroyed after due authorization. Generally, reprocessing is permitted only if it is sure to produce a product that will meet the same quality requirements after the re-working. Reprocessed batch details must be carefully monitored throughout their shelf life and the records must indicate the identity as a reprocessed batch.

12.4 WASTE DISPOSAL

Pharmaceutical industry generates a lot of waste during the manufacturing and testing of drugs. It is important to ensure that this waste is appropriately treated to prevent it from polluting the environment.

According to the provisions of cGMP under Schedule M of the Drugs & Cosmetics Act,

1. Sewage and effluents from a pharmaceutical manufacturing unit must conform with regulations of the Environment Pollution Control Board.

2. All bio-medical waste destruction should proceed in keeping with the provisions of the Bio-Medical Waste (Management and Handling) Rules, 1996.

3. Rejected drugs must be stored and disposed with extra care to prevent them from getting mixed up with stock meant for distribution.

4. Waste disposal records shall be maintained.

5. Materials awaiting disposal must be stored in a safe way to avoid their misuse, and also to prevent any cross-contamination or mixups.

12.4.1 Types of Waste

Waste in the pharmaceutical industry may be of different types, and it generally falls into the following categories:

1. Hazardous wastes
2. Non-hazardous wastes
3. Inert substances
4. Biomedical wastes

(a) Hazardous wastes: As the name indicates, these are wastes that are potentially dangerous to human health or the environment. They may be solid, liquids, gas-containing or sludgy in nature. Such waste contains chemical products that may be ignitable (example-inflammable organic solvents), corrosive (example-strong acids and alkalis), reactive (example-fumes, gases) and toxic (example-heavy metals).

(b) Non-hazardous wastes: These are materials that do not present a significant hazard at the levels in which they are present.

(c) Inert substances: These are materials that do not have any therapeutic effect, but they are used for supportive nutrition, for example, dextrose or sodium chloride solutions. They may however become mixed with other chemicals and therefore, have to be checked for hazardous properties before further disposal.

(d) Biomedical wastes: These are wastes generated during treatment or diagnosis of human beings or animals, or during biological material production and testing. Hospital waste is a major example of this type.

12.4.2 Disposal of Pharmaceutical Waste

Several methods of disposal may be used in pharmaceutical waste management.

1. Incineration or thermal treatment:

In this method, solid organic waste materials are incinerated or burnt to convert them into gaseous products and a solid residue in the form of ash. This is one of the most effective methods, and can be used for disposal of solid, liquid as well as gaseous wastes. While there are mixed opinions on its dangers such as emission of polluting gases, it is certainly one of the best ways to dispose hazardous wastes such as biomedical waste.

This method is unsuitable for wastes that are highly reactive chemicals containing halogens, halogenated plastics, mercury, pressurized gases and radiographic waste.

The ash produced after incineration must be disposed into a secure landfill. There must be arrangements to prevent gases produced during the combustion process from causing air pollution.

2. Chemical disinfection:

This method involves treating waste materials with some chemicals that will inactivate the chemicals or biological materials that may be present in liquid waste. The effectiveness of the process depends on the type of chemical used, its concentration, and nature of contact between the disinfectant material and the wastes.

3. Microwaving:

Microwaving involves the use of microwave radiation and can destroy the infectious materials in biomedical waste. It is advantageous because the electricity requirement is less; steam is not needed either. However, it is not very suitable for pharmaceutical waste. Also, waste must be shredded prior to microwaving in order to allow the radiation to come into contact with the waste material.

4. Autoclaving:

Here, saturated steam is passed through the waste in the autoclave for a duration and at a temperature sufficient to destroy pathogens. This is most commonly used for biomedical waste disposal and also waste generated from the microbiological testing laboratory. The waste produced after autoclaving must be disposed by landfilling. Autoclaving is not the best method for chemical or pharmaceutical waste.

5. Secure land filling:

Here, the wastes are disposed by burying in a landfill that has been designed to contain the hazardous wastes. Unless properly designed and operated, the landfill may lead to liquid leaching into the ground water, attraction of vermin and other such problems. It is also important to have gas extraction systems in the landfills to remove the carbon dioxide and methane that get produced by the anerobic breakdown of waste.

6. Deep burial:

In this method, waste is buried in deep pits or trenches that are at least 2 metres deep. One must ensure the soil is impermeable in these areas, and that there are no shallow wells in the area to avoid the risk of water contamination. Half the pit is covered with the biomedical waste, and rest is filled with lime, stopping 50 cm below the ground surface. The final layer of the pit is made up of soil to cover the waste. Such burial should be done only in areas that are not prone to flooding.

7. Waste encapsulation – immobilization:

Encapsulation of waste involves making waste immobile in the form of a solid block contained within a steel or plastic drum. Clean drums are filled to 75% of their capacity with waste; the remaining space is filled with either cement or lime-cement mix, or bituminous sand or plastic foam. The drum is then sealed and placed at the bottom of a landfill and fresh solid waste if covered on top of it.

8. Waste immobilization – inertization:

Inertization involves grinding of pharmaceutical products after removing them from the packing materials. The ground product is mixed with cement, water and lime and made into a paste. This paste is transported to a landfill and poured into normal waste where it sets as a solid mass.

9. Sewer treatment:

Liquid drug products can be largely diluted by mixing with water and flushed down the sewer very slowly in small quantities. Small quantities of very diluted medicines may be flushed down fast flowing water bodies too.

12.4.3 Effluent Treatment of Pharmaceutical Waste

Pharmaceutical waste water usually contains active pharmaceutical ingredients, excipients, solvents, chemicals, grease and oil. It must be therefore treated in the right way to remove the toxic materials and avoid pollution of ground water or other water bodies in the area.

An effluent treatment plant consists of the following mode of treatment

1. Preliminary treatment through filters to remove particulate matter and floating solids, and allow only waste water to enter the collection tank.

2. Aeration of collected water which then flows to neutralization tank.

3. Adjustment of pH of water to neutral level (pH 6 to 7) by adding lime or aluminium bisulphate, and then water is pumped into settling tank.

4. Flocculation and coagulation is achieved by addition of alum and polyelectrolyte solutions with continuous aeration. Coagulated material in the form of sludge settles at the bottom of the tank, and effluent is sent to the septic tank.

5. Addition of nutrients to septic tank to promote growth of bacteria that will bring about biological degradation of organic materials present in the effluent. Sludge produced is again separated and effluent is sent to activated carbon filter to remove any coloring matter.

6. Clear, treated waste water that is obtained may be used for irrigation of plants on the premises.

REVIEW QUESTIONS

1. What is a product complaint? Which are the different types of complaints?
2. Explain the handling of product complaints.
3. List out the important information that must be present in a product complaint data sheet.
4. Describe voluntary and statutory recall of drug products.
5. Discuss the CDSCO classification of drug recalls.
6. Name any 3 major drug recalls in history, and explain the reasons for these recalls.
7. Describe Schedule M requirements for waste disposal of pharmaceuticals.
8. Classify types of waste.
9. Explain any 3 methods of waste disposal of medicines.
10. List out the steps in effluent treatment in a pharmaceutical facility.

☝ ☝ ☝

Chapter ... 13

DOCUMENTATION IN PHARMACEUTICAL INDUSTRY

Objectives:

Upon completion of this section, the student should be able to

- Enumerate the importance of documentation in the pharmaceutical industry
- Explain good documentation practices to be followed
- Classify the document types
- Define the terms Master Formula Record, Batch Manufacturing Record and Standard Operating Procedure
- Explain how to write an SOP
- List some of the common SOPs that need to be present in a pharmaceutical unit
- Define the term quality review and quality audit
- List different quality documents to be maintained and their contents
- Explain the significance of distribution records

Introduction

On 7th March, 1972, newspapers in the United Kingdom reported news of a shocking disaster where 5 people died from non-sterile dextrose infusions. A government enquiry revealed the cause to be improper sterilization due to which the dextrose infusions became contaminated and caused sepsis in patients who received the non-sterile infusions. What had actually happened was that the autoclave was not properly maintained and would often malfunction. Operators, who did not fully understand the critical nature of the autoclaving process, would deviate from the operating instructions, leading to a faulty process and failure of sterilization, which caused this mishap.

This event, known as the Devonport Incident, was the trigger that created awareness of the need for process and equipment validation. It also highlighted the importance of written instructions, and making sure every person involved with a particular process is made aware of the need to follow the written instructions without any unauthorized modifications.

13.1 IMPORTANCE OF DOCUMENTATION IN PHARMACEUTICAL INDUSTRY

Proper documentation is the backbone of current Good Manufacturing Practices (cGMP) and in the regulatory world, it is commonly held that "If it isn't documented, it wasn't done!"

Documentation is the most essential part of a quality management and quality assurance system for the following reasons:

- Documents are evidence of all manufacturing and testing activities and provide traceability to verify if certain actions were performed or not.
- Written procedures provide clarity and ensure there are no errors that may arise during spoken communication.
- Records, documents and reports give a clear picture of what has been done and is ongoing work, and it also helps to plan better for the future.
- A comprehensive review of the documents maintained in a pharmaceutical facility is often the key used by regulatory bodies to assess the quality function of the facility.
- Accurate and clear records allow the critical reviewing of processes, which can help to improve quality and create cost-saving measures too.
- Good documentation is a must to attain ISO certification and any other industry-specific certifications.

13.2 GOOD DOCUMENTATION PRACTICES

- Documents must be designed and prepared with care. They must be accurate and written in a way that ensures consistency and prevents any errors.
- Content in the documents must be unambiguous. All documents must have a title, nature, and purpose must be clearly stated. Content must be arranged in an orderly manner and allow for easy checking.
- Full text spellings must be used the first time, with the abbreviation in brackets. Subsequently, abbreviations may be used in the rest of the document.
- All documents must carry an effective date, and review date if applicable.
- All documents must be approved; they must bear the signature (with date) of the persons preparing, reviewing and approving the document.
- All documents must have a distinct identification number and version number.
- Documents must be reviewed periodically and in case of revision, the version number must change. Only the most current version must be available; systems must exist to prevent the use of documents that have been superseded.
- No document must be handwritten. However, there may be provision for entry of data by hand (for example, in the Batch Manufacturing Record, where real-time data entries are made). Sufficient space must be available for making the entries, which must be made with indelible ink in a legible manner. Using temporary recording on scraps of paper etc. is totally prohibited.

- If a correction is to be made to a record/entry, it must be made in such a way that the original information is not defaced. Overwriting and use of white ink or correction fluid or sticky notes to make corrections is prohibited; however, it is acceptable to strike through the incorrect entry with a single line, and write the correct entry next to it. The correction must be accompanied by a signature/initial and dated. Where necessary, the reason why the correction has been made must also be recorded such as 'typographical error' or 'calculation error' or 'recording error'.

- Entries in the record must be made immediately – that is, at the time of the particular action.

- Signature and date must accompany the entry where specified. No person should sign for another staff unless specifically authorized. Forging of initials or signatures is prohibited.

- Master copies of documents must be stored securely. Only authorized persons must have access to these. Copies may be made for issuing; while handing over the copies, details have to be recorded of who issued the document, to whom, and the date and time of issue.

- Copies reproduced from master documents must be clear enough to allow comprehension.

- If printouts are obtained on thermal paper from an instrument, they must be photocopied (as the print will fade over time). Both the original and photocopy labeled as "Copy of original" must be attached to the report.

- Critical records must be stored securely, protected against loss, falsification or any damage by the elements, with limited access to only authorized persons.

- Copies of critical records must be available in electronic form or paper or microfilm and be stored separate from the originals.

- In case of electronic data processing methods, access to the master templates and documents must be given only to authorized persons to enter data or modify it in the computer. Passwords and biometrics may be used to control access.

- If electronic signatures are to be used, they must be unique to the person. Such electronic signature is generally by means of an identification code which comprises a username and password. Using saved digital image of the hand-written signature of the person is not permitted.

- Retaining of important documents (such as developmental history, technical reports, validation reports, production and control records, training records, distribution records etc.) must be done in keeping with regulatory requirements. For example, records about the production, testing and distribution of a batch of drug product must be retained for a minimum of 1 year following the expiry date of that batch.

Common Documentation Errors

1. Illegible entries.
2. Falsified data (date/time/version number).
3. Signatures missing.
4. Raw data to support results missing.
5. Missing documents.
6. Discarding data that does not match requirements.
7. Invalid and fabricated data.
8. No recording of activities.
9. Data manipulation/deletion.
10. Incomplete records.

Excerpt from a warning letter issued by USFDA to a firm citing lack of adequate documentation practices.

"...Your quality unit (QU) lacks appropriate responsibility and control over your drug manufacturing operations.

During the inspection, our investigator observed discarded cGMP documents and evidence of uncontrolled shredding of documents. For example, multiple bags of uncontrolled cGMP documents with color coding indicating they were from drug production, quality, and laboratory operations were awaiting shredding. Our investigator also found a blue binder containing cGMP records, including batch records for U.S. drug products, discarded with other records in a 55-gallon drum in your scrap yard. CGMP documents in the binder were dated as recently as January 21, 2019: seven days before our inspection. Your QU did not review or check these documents prior to disposal...."

"...The uncontrolled destruction of cGMP records, and your lack of adequate documentation practices, raise questions about the effectiveness of your QU and the integrity and accuracy of your cGMP records...."

"...Your quality system does not adequately ensure the accuracy and integrity of data to support the safety, effectiveness, and quality of the drugs you manufacture..."

13.3 TYPES OF DOCUMENTS

The records and documents in the pharmaceutical industry are categorized into the following classes:

1. Primary records (contracts, production formulae, packing instructions, supply source documents etc.).
2. Procedures or supporting documents (SOPs, instructions, manuals, guidebooks).
3. Subsidiary records (equipment/instrument printouts, calibration reading reports etc.).
4. Quality control records (test methods, test results, investigations, internal audit reports, Corrective and Preventive Action (CAPA) reports, recall files etc.).

Commonly Used Documents

Document name	Description
Quality manual	Describes the regulations (USFDA/Schedule M/ ICH/ WHO) the company must follow to achieve desired level of compliance with cGMP in all operations and products.
Company policy	General description of company's outlook on different aspects of the company's business and their implementation.
Standard Operating Procedures (SOPs)	Stepwise instructions to perform a given task.
Batch records	Stepwise instruction for production and packaging of drug product. Include records relating to each batch, and contain entries made during these processes.
Logbooks	Bound books or collection of forms in which operation, maintenance and calibration details of equipment is recorded.
Specifications	List of requirements that materials and products must meet to be considered acceptable.
Test methods	Stepwise instructions for testing of materials and products.

13.4 MASTER FORMULA RECORD (MFR)

A Master Formula Record is defined as an approved master document, with instructions of how the entire manufacturing process must be performed for each batch size of each product to be manufactured. This document ensures that there is uniformity across batches of the same product. The MFR must be prepared, signed and dated by one competent individual, and independently checked, signed and dated by another competent person in the quality department. All processing of a given batch must proceed as per its MFR.

Contents of MFR:

- Name of product, its strength and dosage form description.
- Name and measure/weight of each active ingredient per dosage unit or per unit weight or per measure of drug product.
- Statement of total weight or measure of a dosage unit.
- List of component names and their weight or measure using same weight system.
- Statement of theoretical weight or measure where necessary in the processing phase.

- Statement of theoretical yield with minimum and maximum percentage of yield acceptable beyond which there must be an investigation of the process.
- Description of containers, closures and packaging materials to be used for the drug product packing.
- Specimen or copy of each label/labeling material with date and signature of authorized person who has approved the labeling.
- All manufacturing and control instructions in detail.
- Procedures for sampling and testing.
- Specifications for raw materials, intermediates and finished products.
- Instructions for storage of intermediates and finished products.
- Special notations and precautions to be observed.

13.5 BATCH MANUFACTURING RECORD (BMR)

Also known sometimes as the Batch Production Record, this is an approved copy of the MFR for each batch of product being processed, in which data has been filled in during processing of the batch. It contains details of location where production is done, data entries, names of operators making the entries and their signatures with dates, supporting data records (such as cleaning records, equipment calibration details, in-process and final quality control test reports etc).

The BMR bears details of the unique batch number assigned to that particular batch. This information must be recorded in a log book along with date on which batch number is allotted, the identity of the product and the batch size.

Contents of BMR

- Name of the product.
- Date and time of commencement and completion of important stages in the processing.
- Name of persons responsible for each critical stage, with initials of operators handling each operation and persons who checked these operations.
- Name and quantities of each raw material actually weighed with the batch number from which the material was drawn (including details of any re-processed materials added).
- Major equipment used in the processing.
- Results of readings for critical processing parameters.
- Details of samples drawn.

- In-process testing reports.

- Actual yield obtained at critical phases.

- Any deviations from procedure, with signatures to authorize the deviations; their evaluation and investigation if conducted.

- Packaging material and label description, with representative material attached.

- Results and reports of QC testing of final product for approval of the batch.

- Statement about decision taken regarding approval or rejection of the batch along with the date, and name and signature of person making this decision.

Data Recording in Logbooks

- Logbooks must be maintained for critical production equipment, analytical instruments and for environmental conditions in areas where processing takes place.

- Entries must be made in chronological order, with dates, at the time of the activity; pre-completion of entries is prohibited.

- Person who performed the operation must be identified.

- Only trained and authorized persons must do the data entry in the logbooks.

- Data recorded must reflect actual display on the equipment panels (for example: with all decimals, no rounding off unless pre-defined and documented instructions exist for this).

- Any unusual observations must also be recorded with date and signature, and immediately reported to personnel in-charge of that area as well as QA department.

- Data which is repeated must be written again; putting –"- marks, or –do – or "Ditto" or "same as above" is not acceptable.

13.6 STANDARD OPERATING PROCEDURE (SOP)

A standard operating procedure (SOP) is a written set of instructions describing step-wise how a routine activity is to be performed. When the SOP is followed exactly, it ensures consistency of the operation being performed exactly as desired, and this makes sure that the desired quality is attained.

An SOP must contain a straightforward description of the task to be carried out, in simple language, and cover all the major steps in performing the task. SOP must be written by persons who have sufficient knowledge and experience with the task being described.

SOPs must be written in clear language using the active tense. (For example, "Switch on the equipment.." and not "The equipment is switched on..."

SOP must be detailed enough to allow someone with even limited knowledge or experience with the task, to perform the task as desired without any supervision. However, it must not involve unnecessarily length descriptions. For example, in some processing SOP, if equipment operation is involved, and that procedure is a very long one, and is clearly available in the equipment operating manual, that procedure may just be referenced in the SOP instead of repeating all those instructions in the SOP.

Any abbreviations or acronyms used in the SOP must be explained at the beginning of the SOP.

SOPs must be prepared by the respective departments, and then reach QA for a review for checking if it complies with cGMP. After QA approval, the SOP must be signed, dated and authorized for issue by senior personnel of the concerned department.

If a need is felt to amend or change any particular in an existing SOP being used, it must go through the change control procedure specified as part of QA.

Contents of SOP:

- Title page
- Table of contents
- Procedures
    - Scope
    - Method summary
    - Definitions
    - Health and safety warnings
    - Cautions
    - Interferences
    - Personnel qualification/responsibility
    - Equipment / supplies
    - Procedure in steps
    - Calibration/standardization
    - Sample collection, handling and preservation
    - Troubleshooting
    - Data entry, calculation and report writing
- QA/QC section
- References section

Common SOPs in a manufacturing unit:

- Organization and personnel
  - Personnel qualifications and experience
  - Personnel hygiene, responsibilities, movement control
  - Personnel training
- Facilities and equipment
  - Facility safety procedures
  - Facility maintenance and cleaning
  - Qualification and validation of critical systems (examples – water system, HVAC etc.)
  - Equipment cleaning and maintenance; log books
  - Qualification of equipment
- Materials management
  - Receiving and storage of materials
  - Sampling of materials
  - Control of accepted and rejected materials
  - Warehousing of finished products
  - Distribution of approved products
- Production
  - Work instructions
  - Operation of equipment
  - All production processes
  - All packing processes
  - BMR entry and checking
  - Personnel safety
  - Control of contamination and cross-contamination
  - Process deviations reports and investigation
  - Control of packaging and labeling
- Quality Assurance
  - Document control, including SOPs
  - MFR and BMR
  - Process validations
  - Review of batch records and batch release
  - Change control
  - GMP training
  - Corrective and Preventive Action (CAPA)

- Quality Control
  - Laboratory safety
  - Analytical methods
  - Sampling and testing of in-process and final goods
  - Calibration of analytical equipment/instruments
  - Maintenance of analytical equipment/instruments
  - Analytical method validation
  - Environmental monitoring
  - Approval or rejection of materials
  - Investigation of Out of Specifications (OOS) results
  - Stability testing

13.7 QUALITY REVIEW

The USFDA requires that quality standards of each drug product must be evaluated at least once a year. Other regulatory bodies have similar requirements and these can be met through the performance of an annual Quality Review.

Annual product quality review is the evaluation of a given product's quality to verify that the existing processes used in its manufacture are consistently producing the desired quality product. This helps to ensure that current specifications for that drug product are adequate; the trends revealed by the data also provide insights for any changes to be introduced in either the manufacturing or control procedures or in the product specifications.

A representative number of batches must be selected, and a review must be done of the documents associated with them to check for adherence to specifications. Both approved and rejected batches must be a part of this study. Along with this, it is also important to evaluate any complaints received regarding the same product batches, or any returns or recalls that have been associated with those batches.

By doing these activities, it is possible to find areas where improvement is necessary. When such improvements are introduced into the next batch being manufactured, it leads to a process that is better capable of manufacturing products of the desired quality.

Quality review includes:

- Starting materials
- Packaging materials
- Critical in-process controls
- Critical equipment qualifications
- Finished product test results
- Stability studies
- Change control procedures
- CAPA effectiveness

- Returns/recalls
- Market complaints
- Deviations/non-conformances
- Failed batches
- Previous batches review

Typically, in a quality review, historical data from batches of a particular product manufactured over the past 12 months is reviewed and analyzed using statistical techniques. This helps to assess if the process is in control or not and if any changes are necessary. Based on the results of the review, re-validation or CAPA may be undertaken.

Following a review of all relevant headings, the higher management must highlight the major observations made, and arrive at conclusions regarding quality improvement. The inferences drawn must result in appropriate recommendations on any corrective actions that may be necessary such as a formulation or packaging change, or revision of specifications, or making processes more robust.

Performing a quality review is vital because it enables the better understanding of processes and this can guide further quality improvements. Such a review also serves as a method of continued process verification. The trends observed in the quality review can be an indication of areas of potential risk; thus, this exercise is also a part of the risk management plan of the company that is recommended by ICH guidelines.

13.8 QUALITY AUDITS

A quality audit is an independent evaluation performed to review if activities are performed in a manner to comply with set objectives defined in the company's quality system. In the pharmaceutical industry, audits are an effective means of verifying if the different departments comply with cGMP regulations.

Purpose of the Audit:

Audits serve to verify if the production and control systems are operating as intended. They help to uncover problem areas and thus, allow the timely correction of issues. Regular audits help to provide confidence that the organization is functioning under effective control. Audits performed in problem situations such as product recall or repeated market complaints is useful to identify non-compliance with cGMP and to drive initiatives to take the necessary corrective actions.

Audit Types:

Quality audits may be of three types – internal audits or self-inspections, external audits for contract manufacturing/testing and regulatory audits performed by regulatory bodies.

Internal audits are done by auditors within the company to assess cGMP compliance, identify problem areas and take corrective action, and to prepare for audits by regulatory bodies.

External audits are carried out by a company at the sites of its vendors or contract manufacturers or testing laboratories. This type of audit helps to assess if the outside party understands the contract-giver's requirements and adheres to the quality system to reduce failure risk.

Regulatory audits are performed by regulatory bodies to check for adherence to statutory requirements. These audits are a must to ensure data quality and integrity in respect of products that seek regulatory approval.

After completion of the audit, an audit report is prepared with complete details of the areas audited, and the deficiencies observed. The report also suggests which corrective actions are required to remove problem areas, and for improvement of the quality system.

13.9 QUALITY DOCUMENTATION

This comprises all the documents that form part of the company's quality management system. This includes documents such as the quality policy, quality procedures, work instructions and records. These documents are arranged in a definite hierarchy based on their scope.

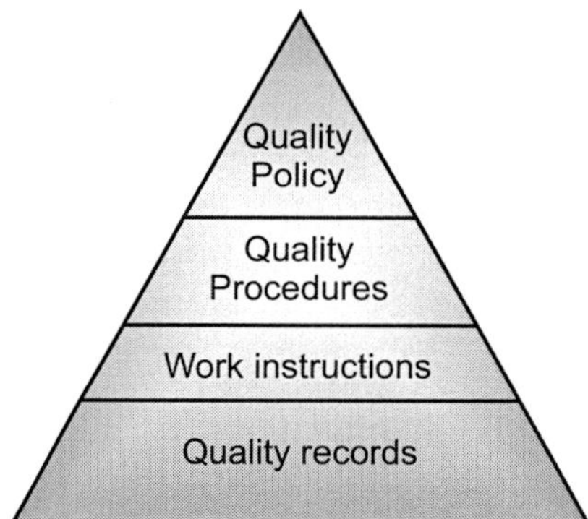

Fig. 13.1: Quality Documentation Pyramid

Quality policy/ Manual: Describes the quality system and what is to be done as an organization to implement it. Also answers the question of why this quality system is being implemented. In the pharmaceutical industry, this part will include the regulations to be followed by the company such as USFDA guidelines/ICH guidelines/Schedule M requirements/WHO-GMP requirements etc.

Quality Procedures: Describes how the quality system will be implemented, methods to be used, who should do what, when, and where. More detailed than policy document.

Work Instructions: Specific to departments, and spell out details of how each task is to be done. Detailed instructions are given, and may include diagrams, job sheets etc. In the pharma industry, this is represented by SOPs.

Records: Evidence documents that prove that quality policy, procedures and work instructions have been implemented as directed. In the pharmaceutical field, this includes batch manufacturing records, QC test reports, validation documents etc.

13.10 DISTRIBUTION RECORDS

Batches are released for distribution by the QC department only after thorough testing and approval. The warehousing department must maintain records of batches released for distribution in a systematic manner. For every batch of product, it is important to maintain distribution records in sufficient detail to be able to trace to which places the product has been sent. This is critical in the event of a problem with the product batch that necessitates a product recall from the market.

Distribution record details:

Some of the important details required include:

- Name of the product, its strength, and description of dosage form.

- Batch number/lot number of shipped product.

- Name and address of consignee.

- Shipping date and quantity shipped.

- Besides warehouse inventory records, distribution records also include invoices, receipts from customers and bill of lading.

The February 28, 2019 edition of Pharma Times Now provides a review of data collected regarding the "Top 20 Reasons for Drug Recalls in the USA". The topmost category cited is the violation of cGMP which was the cause for the highest number of recalls – 238. In the pharmaceutical industry, compliance with cGMP is the basic quality requirement that ensures the production of safe and effective medicines. While there is increasing awareness of the need to adopt quality systems, the pharmaceutical industry still has a long way to go to make sure all personnel involved in the manufacturing of drug products understand the criticality of following practices as laid down in the written documents of the company.

REVIEW QUESTIONS

1. Write a note on the significance of documentation in pharmaceutical industry.

2. Explain important guidelines of Good Documentation Practices.

3. List measures to be taken for electronic documentation systems.

4. Define MFR, BMR and SOP.

5. Describe the contents of an SOP.

6. Discuss the significance of logbooks and how they must be used for data recording.

7. Write a standard operating procedure for "Writing an SOP".

8. What is a quality review and how is it different from quality audit?

9. Name and describe the quality-related documents to be maintained in a pharmaceutical company.

Case Studies – Refer to https://www.igmpiindia.org/DocumentationandMaintenance.pdf

Chapter ...14

CALIBRATION AND VALIDATION

Objectives:

Upon completion of this section, the student should be able to

- Define the terms calibration, qualification and validation in the pharmaceutical industry.
- Explain the significance of calibration, qualification and validation.
- Outline the phases of qualification.
- Describe the different types of validation – prospective, concurrent and retrospective.
- Define and explain Validation Master Plan (VMP).
- Explain the conditions that necessitate revalidation.
- Define analytical method validation and important parameters to be validated.

Introduction

The pharmaceutical industry is driven by the need for safe and effective products that are of the desired quality. Quality assurance is a concept that emphasizes building quality into products. For this to be achieved, it is vital that all components that are part of the manufacturing and testing process must perform as expected, and provide results that are accurate, precise and reliable. Measuring instruments and other equipment and tools used at different stages must therefore be capable of providing accurate data. Any change in their performance characteristics may lead to costly errors that may even pose a danger to life. Calibration and validation are two aspects that help to avoid such errors and ensure a quality product reaches the patient.

14.1 CALIBRATION

Even a small error during manufacture or packing or storage of a pharmaceutical product can have a severe impact on the health of thousands of patients who consume it. This is the reason why regulatory bodies lay down stringent quality parameters that pharma companies must meet to get their products approved. Measurement of these parameters at different stages in the manufacture of drugs is done using several instruments. Naturally, it follows that the ability of these instruments to provide accurate measurements is critical to the manufacturing process. Assessing this ability is the very purpose of the activity called CALIBRATION.

14.1.1 Definition

Calibration is defined as the process of determining the accuracy of an instrument. This involves:

(a) Obtaining a particular reading from the instrument under study.

(b) Comparing this reading with one obtained from a standard instrument.

(c) Assessing the degree of variation between the two readings.

(d) Adjusting the instrument so that it gives readings in keeping with established standards.

14.1.2 Objectives of Calibration

Calibration of an instrument helps to assess its accuracy. It helps to determine how accurately the instrument is producing results within the prescribed limits.

The main purposes of calibration are:

1. To ensure instrument/equipment readings display correct readings each time.

2. To determine how accurate, precise and reliable are the measurements produced, as well as the degree of deviations that are produced.

3. To check how reliable the instrument is by examining if it delivers reproducible results.

4. To assess the degree of drift from accuracy over time.

5. To ensure adherence to cGMP guidelines for quality.

When an instrument has to be calibrated, its measurements are compared with the ones obtained from a standard instrument. Comparison may also be made against an existing instrument that is known to give measurements at a level exceeding the prescribed limits of accuracy and precision. Generally, the accuracy of the standard must be ten times that of the instrument under test. However, an accuracy ratio of 3 : 1 is also acceptable by regulatory authorities.

14.1.3 Significance of Calibration

When instruments and equipment are used regularly, over time, they tend to undergo some or the other damage. This results in a shift in the measurement so that the devices are no longer giving accurate and precise results over the expected range. By measuring the accuracy, precision and range of such devices, calibration helps to track the shifts and the data generated can be used to rectify the functioning of the instrument.

Sometimes, ambient conditions such as humidity, temperature and pressure may cause a drift in the measurements made by instruments. Calibrating such instruments at regular intervals can help to ensure the drift does not exceed acceptable limits.

Thus, regular calibration of equipment and instruments makes it possible to guarantee that they continue to function without any error and in turn, this ensures reproducible pharmaceutical quality of the products.

When calibration is not done for a long time, it may lead to:
- Faulty measurements and discrepancies that impact final product quality.
- Deterioration of drug materials leading to a safety threat to those consuming the product.
- Waste of resources and time.
- Loss of time because of faulty process which has to be shut down and re-started after calibration.
- Product recall because of damaged drug products.

14.1.4 Frequency of Calibration

The frequency of instrument calibration depends on the nature of its variation or drift from accuracy over time. It also depends on how important that particular instrument's measurement is to determine the quality of the end product. It is therefore important to set up a calibration schedule for each instrument such as weekly, monthly, bi-monthly, quarterly, half-yearly or annually. Generally, instruments need to be calibrated in the following situations:

1. As soon as it is installed, before it is used for the first time.
2. Both before and after taking any measurement that is critical to product quality.
3. When anything out of the ordinary occurs – for example, a fall, bump, or electrical shock is generated.
4. When readings appear suspect in accuracy.
5. After any repair work has been done on the instrument.
6. As part of routine calibration schedule.
7. At all those times recommended by the instrument manufacturer.

14.1.5 Calibration Methods

Instruments can be calibrated in several different ways. The method chosen generally depends on what results one desires from the calibration exercise and also on particular regulatory requirements that are to be met. The three common procedures used for calibration include - Standard Calibration, ISO 17025 Accredited Calibration, and Calibration with Data.

Calibration plays a vital role in controlling the uncertainty around process measurements. Regular calibration can reduce errors, improve accuracy of instruments and make it easier to ensure good quality of the final product. Thus, it is vital for pharmaceutical companies to have a calibration schedule that will give them confidence in their process measurement and control.

14.2 QUALIFICATION

Just as measuring instruments need to be calibrated, it is important to demonstrate that the equipment and utilities in a pharmaceutical company are appropriate for their intended use, and to prove that they are performing as expected. The activities undertaken to generate such evidence is called as Qualification.

14.2.1 Definition

Qualification may be defined as the act of proving and documenting that a given equipment or process or utility is correctly installed, working properly, and is consistently producing the expected results.

Qualification is a part of the process of validation; however qualification alone does not complete process validation.

14.2.2 Phases of Qualification

There are four major phases of qualification – Design Qualification (DQ), Installation Qualification (IQ), Operational Qualification (OQ) and Performance Qualification (PQ).

(a) Design Qualification is defined as documented verification that the proposed design of equipment, systems and facilities is appropriate for the intended purpose. DQ must be performed whenever purchasing new equipment; it should also be performed when existing equipment is going to be used for any new application.

(b) Installation Qualification is defined as documented evidence that the equipment, supporting utilities and premises have been built or installed in keeping with design specifications. IQ serves to verify that equipment installation has been done as recommended by the manufacturer, in the correct manner, and kept in a suitable environment.

(c) Operational Qualification is defined as establishing documented evidence that an equipment, facility or utilities functions as intended, in keeping with its operational specifications. OQ thus helps to verify that the installed equipment works correctly.

(d) Performance Qualification is defined as establishing documented evidence that the process works to consistently produce a product that meets all the predetermined quality requirements. PQ helps to verify that performance within the specified limits is as expected.

WHO Definitions

DQ - Documented evidence that the premises, supporting systems, utilities, equipment and processes have been designed in accordance with the requirements of good manufacturing practices.

IQ - The performance of tests to ensure that the installations (such as machines, measuring devices, utilities and manufacturing areas) used in a manufacturing process are appropriately selected and correctly installed and operate in accordance with established specifications.

OQ - Documented verification that the system or subsystem performs as intended over all anticipated operating ranges.

PQ - Documented verification that the equipment or system operates consistently and gives reproducibility within defined specifications and parameters for prolonged periods.

Scope of Qualification Phases

Phase of qualification	Question it answers
Design qualification	Has it been designed (or selected) correctly?
Installation qualification	Has it been installed (or built) correctly?
Operational qualification	Is it working correctly?
Performance qualification	Is it performing correctly within specified limits?

14.2.3 Considerations While Doing Qualification

The following factors must be considered when doing qualification:

1. Qualification must be performed as per predetermined and approved qualification protocols.
2. Results must be recorded and should be a part of the qualification reports.
3. Areas or rooms must be qualified before utilities; utilities must be qualified before equipment.
4. Equipment can be used only after it has been qualified and documented evidence shows that it is suitable for the intended purpose.
5. Qualification should be done in a logical sequence – first DQ, then IQ, then OQ and finally PQ.
6. Some stages of qualification may be performed by a third party; however, the final responsibility of ensuring the qualification is done as per GMP rests with the contract-giver.
7. All documents related to the qualification process (specifications, standard operating procedures, manuals, acceptance criteria and certificates) should be maintained.
8. All equipment, utilities and systems must be maintained in a qualified state at all times. When necessary, they must undergo periodic requalification.
9. Validation of processes must be done using qualified equipment only.

14.2.4 Requalification

When any equipment undergoes any kind of modification or relocation on a scale that has a direct impact on the product quality, it must undergo a re-qualification. This process must be handled with a documented change control procedure, after due review and authorization.

14.2.5 Factory Acceptance Test and Site Acceptance Test

In some situations, equipment, or a system or utility may be assembled fully or partially at some other site. In such cases, testing and verification must be performed to ensure it is fit for dispatch, and results must be recorded in the Factory Acceptance Test report before shipment of the item.

After the shipment is received by the end user, tests must be repeated to verify that the equipment or system or utility is of acceptable quality. Results of these tests must be recorded in the Site Acceptance Test report.

14.3 VALIDATION

Every pharmaceutical manufacturer has to comply with the requirements of current Good Manufacturing Practices (cGMP). In order to verify that quality standards are being met, there has to be a systematic approach by which data is collected and studied to confirm that processes operate as intended. This systematic approach is called as Validation.

When a process is validated, it ensures a high level of assurance that batches produced by that same process will be uniform and meet pre-determined quality requirements. Thus, validation serves to confirm that a given process has been developed correctly and that it operates within specific controls. In turn, this assures that quality products are being consistently produced and reduces the chances of rejected batches and the need for reworking. In other words, a validated process offers a significant cost reduction as compared to processes running without validation.

Worldwide, validation is now considered an integral part of Good Manufacturing Practices. A manufacturer who wishes to get approval to manufacture drugs or to introduce new drug products into the market must comply with validation requirements as specified by regulatory bodies.

It is important to remember that validation is not a one-off process, it is part of an ongoing activity to ensure that quality products are consistently produced.

14.3.1 History of Validation

In the mid-1970s, several issues were encountered in sterility of large volume parenterals. In response to this, two FDA officials, Bud Loftus and Ted Byers proposed the concept of validation in order to avoid such quality issues. Initially, validation activities were centred around the processes involved in this category of products; later, the idea spread to other areas of the pharmaceutical industry. Thus, validation was a concept pioneered by the US FDA. However, there was no definition or mention of it in the regulations until 1978.

14.3.2 Definition

Each of the regulatory bodies have defined validation in different words. Some of the important definitions include:

European Commission, 1991:

"Validation is the act of proving, in accordance with GMPs, that any process actually leads to the expected results."

In 2000, this definition was modified to read as:

"Validation is documented evidence that the process, operated within established Parameters, can perform effectively and reproducibly to produce a Medicinal product meeting its predetermined specifications and quality attributes."

US FDA Definition:

"Process validation is establishing documented evidence which provides a high degree of assurance that a specified process will consistently produce a product meeting its pre-determined specifications and quality characteristics."

ICH Definition:

"Process Validation is the means of ensuring and providing documentary evidence that processes within their specified design parameters are capable of repeatedly and reliably producing a finished product of the required quality."

WHO Definition:

"Validation is the documented act of proving that any procedure, process, equipment, material, activity or system actually leads to expected result."

14.3.3 Scope of Validation

Pharmaceutical manufacturers have to make sure their validation program covers all the important areas of pharmaceutical processing. The major areas include:

- Equipment validation (also called qualification).
- Facilities and utilities validation (water system, air handling unit, compressed gas system, computer systems).
- Process validation.
- Cleaning validation.
- Analytical method validation.
- Instrument calibration.

Validation needs to be carried out for any new equipment, premises, utilities, systems, procedures, processes. It must also be performed when any major change has occurred in any of these. Validation is different from in-process tests – the latter only helps in monitoring that a process runs as expected, whereas validation aims at demonstrating that a given process is suitable for routine use because it consistently yields product of desired quality. In this sense, validation activities will focus on the most critical aspects of processes, and these are arrived at through a risk assessment approach.

14.3.4 Advantages of Validation

- Optimized processes.
- Assured quality of products.
- Reduced cost of maintaining quality.
- Increased output.
- Reduced complaints, rejections, batch failure, mix-ups and cross-contamination.
- Faster scale-up from pilot level to manufacturing level.
- Better compliance with regulatory requirements.

14.3.5 Types of Validation

Validation can be done at different stages of the process. Accordingly, there are three main types of validation as follows:

1. Prospective Validation – done before the process commences
2. Concurrent Validation – done as the process is going on
3. Retrospective Validation – done on already completed process

14.3.5.1 Prospective Validation

It is defined as establishing documented evidence that a given system actually does what it purports to do on the basis of a previously determined protocol. This type of validation is generally carried out before the start of a new process of manufacture. It must be done on a minimum of three consecutive batches of the product.

To carry out this validation, each step of the proposed process is evaluated to determine which parameters are critical to the quality of the finished product. With this information, experiments are designed and documented in an authorized protocol.

Prospective validation protocol must cover the evaluation of all the equipment, facilities, utilities and analytical test procedures that will be used in production of the new product. Only after data has been obtained about the critical process parameters, it will be possible to prepare the Master Batch Records.

Using such a well-defined process, a series of product batched must be produced. The number of batch runs to be carried out must be sufficient to allow the collection of data for evaluation. Generally, three consecutive batch runs are considered sufficient for a complete validation of the process. However, in reality, more than three runs may also be required to arrive at sufficiently reliable data.

During a validation run, the batch size must be kept the same as that intended for regular industrial scale production. If it is intended to sell the validation batch products, care must be taken to produce the batches in conditions that comply completely with cGMP (current Good Manufacturing Practices). Also, such batches may be sold only after verifying that the validation exercise has given a satisfactory outcome and been authorized for marketing after passing all quality requirements.

When the validation batches are being processed, samples should be drawn at frequent intervals and tests should be performed at different stages of the production process; all results must be documented thoroughly. Final products in their final packs must also be tested for comprehensive data collection.

When deciding on the validation strategy, it is good to obtain data using different lots of active ingredients and major additives. Batches manufactured during different shifts, using different facilities and equipment that will be used for commercial production, must be evaluated. Readings must be taken over a wide operating range for the most critical operations, and all data obtained must be exhaustively analyzed.

Once the data generated has been reviewed, guidelines can be prepared regarding the level of monitoring necessary as a part of in-process controls during regular production. All such guidelines should be made a part of the Batch Manufacturing Record and Batch Packing Record. If necessary, they must also be added into the relevant Standard Operating Procedures (SOPs).

Prospective validation data is also to be used to determine limits, frequencies of testing, and actions to be taken in situations when the limits are exceeded.

Information in Prospective Validation Protocol

- Brief description of process to be validation.
- Summary of the critical manufacturing steps to be studied.
- List of facilities and equipment to be used including monitoring/recording/measuring instruments/equipment and their calibration status.
- Analytical test methods to be used and their validation status.
- In-process controls proposed and their acceptance criteria.
- Sampling plan and procedures.
- Methods to record results and evaluate the data obtained.
- Specifications for finished product acceptance.
- Additional tests to be performed and their acceptance criteria and validation status.
- Proposed timeframe for validation process.
- Functions and responsibilities in the validation program.

14.3.5.2 Concurrent Validation

Concurrent validation involves monitoring of the critical processing and testing steps at the in-process stage. It is almost the same as prospective validation except that the manufacturer will sell the products manufactured during the validation run, provided they meet all the pre-determined quality requirements. There must be documents maintained that show the justification for a concurrent validation, and due approval of the decision by authorized persons. Documentation for concurrent validation is same as that for prospective validation.

14.3.5.3 Retrospective Validation

Retrospective validation is defined as establishing documented evidence that a system performs as purported, by reviewing the historical data that had been collected during the manufacturing and testing stages. This validation is done for products that have already been distributed; this method of validation is therefore, acceptable, only for processes that are well-established and stabilized over many years of production. Retrospective validation is unsuitable in cases where there has been any recent change in either the product composition, or processing steps, or equipment used in the manufacture and testing of the product.

A specific protocol must be prepared first, outlining the way in which the retrospective validation will be carried out. Historical data is collected from batch manufacturing and packaging records, equipment logbooks, process control charts, personnel change records, finished product testing data, and stability test results. After historical data collection and review, results must be reported, along with a conclusion and recommendations, if any.

Batches for retrospective validation must be selected in a manner to represent all the batches made during the period selected for review. The number of batches included in the validation must be sufficient to prove consistency of the process. Generally, data is collected from anywhere between 10 and 30 consecutive batches. If fewer batches will be used, the reason must be justified and documented. Any batches that did not meet the specifications during the review period, must also be included. In some cases, samples retained after distribution may be tested to obtain necessary data.

Elements to be considered for retrospective validation:

- Batches manufactured during the defined period (ex – 10 last successive batches).
- Batches released per year.
- Batch size and strength.
- Master manufacturing and packaging records.
- Latest specifications for APIs and finished product.
- Process deviations list.
- Corrective actions list.
- Records of manufacturing document changes/revisions.
- Stability testing data for several batches.

14.3.6 Revalidation

During the normal course of operations, it may become necessary to introduce changes in the process for improving the quality. Occasionally, new equipments or instruments may be installed, or there may be a change in the utility systems. Whenever any such changes are introduced, it is vital to prove that these changes do not have any adverse effect on the process or the product quality. Collecting such evidence is described as revalidation. The documentation and other requirements for revalidation match those of prospective validation.

Often, due to wear and tear, over the course of time, there may be a drift from normal operating conditions. This makes it important for manufacturers to make sure they schedule a periodic revalidation of their systems, equipments, facilities and processes to confirm that they continue to perform as expected to meet the prescribed quality requirements.

14.3.6.1 Changes that Necessitate Revalidation

1. Change in raw materials (especially physical properties such as particle size, moisture content, density, viscosity etc. which tend to affect product or process quality.
2. Change in vendor from whom APIs and other raw materials are procured.

3. Change in the primary container or other packaging material.

4. Process changes (such as drying temperature, mixing time, batch size etc.).

5. Substitution of equipment with a new type of equipment (same equipment new model does not require validation; but the qualification steps of DQ, IQ, OQ and PQ must be performed and documented).

6. Any change in the facility/premises/plant.

If a decision is taken to not perform revalidation trials despite a change in the process/equipment, the reason for this decision must be explained and documented.

14.3.7 Validation Master Plan

14.3.7.1 Definition

A Validation Master Plan (VMP) is defined as the document that provides information about the company's validation programme. This document must contain details of validation to be done, and the timeframes for the studies to be performed. There must be clear statements regarding who is responsible for each part of the validation program.

The WHO guidelines define VMP as "A high-level document that establishes and umbrella validation plan for the entire project and summarizes the manufacturer's overall philosophy and approach."

It is important to note the situations in which the words 'validation' and 'qualification' are to be used. When a system or equipment is the focus of the exercise, it is known as 'qualification'.

When a process is the focus of the exercise, it is known as 'validation'.

For example, one may qualify a spray dryer, and validate a drying process; similarly, an autoclave is qualified but the sterilization process is validated.

14.3.7.2 Purpose of VMP

The main purpose of the VMP is to give a comprehensive overview of the complete validation operation, how it has been organized, what all it will cover, and the validation plan.

- It helps to management to understand how much time will be required, personnel to be involved, and expenses expected to be incurred.

- It informs members of the validation team about their jobs and responsibilities.

- It helps inspectors/auditors to understand the company's approach to validation activities.

14.3.7.3 Who should write the VMP?

The best VMP is a result of a team-writing effort because it ensures a representation of the perspectives of different departments involved in the operations. When people from diverse areas of the operation are involved, it is more likely that all possible angles of approaching the VMP are covered. A VMP must be as lengthy as required to convey all the necessary information to ensure a successful validation program.

14.3.7.4 Elements of a Good VMP

Validation Master Plans must contain the following information at the very least:

- Company's validation policy.
- Organizational structure.
- List of items to be validated.
- Brief outline of systems, equipment, facilities and processes to be validated.
- Formats for documenting protocols and test reports.
- Planning and scheduling of validation activities.
- Change control procedure.
- Training requirements for validation team.
- Details of persons responsible for each stage of validation – preparing the plan, drawing up protocols and standard operating procedures (SOPs), actual validation work, preparation and control of reports and documents, approval of validation protocols and reports at every stage of validation, system for tracking validation, training requirements for validation team.

Contents of a VMP:

1. Title page with document number and version information, and authorization in the form of approval signatures.
2. Table of contents listing out critical areas of the VMP.
3. Glossary to define technical terms and abbreviations.
4. Plan for validation – details of the process steps, critical parts of the process that impact product quality and what is to be validated, when, where, how, and why.
5. Management's approach to validation.
6. Scope of the validation – what all will be covered under validation (and what will not be covered too).
7. Roles and responsibilities of the different departments (validation team, manufacturing department, engineering department, Quality Assurance department etc.) for each of the activities involved.
8. Services to be outsourced to outside vendors.
9. Deviation management – how to document, investigate and deal with deviations that may be encountered.
10. Change control procedures.
11. Risk management policy.
12. Training of personnel.
13. Validation matrix that outlines the validation required throughout the manufacturing facility in the order of most to least critical.
14. References – documents that guide the validation process.

14.3.8 Analytical Method Validation

When a raw material, in-process or finished product is tested using certain analytical methods, it is important to confirm that the analytical methods themselves should be producing reliable results. This is ensured by performing validation of analytical methods.

Regulatory requirements too necessitate that test methods used by a company should show sufficient accuracy, specificity, sensitivity and reproducibility. Besides, modern cGMP guidelines require that quality is not merely tested, but built into the product from the very beginning steps. So, it naturally follows that not just the manufacturing steps, but also the analytical methods used for testing products must be designed with certain quality attributes.

14.3.8.1 Definition

Analytical method validation is defined as the process of establishing, through laboratory studies, that the procedure's performance characteristics meet the requirements for its intended use.

Analytical method validation is not a one-time activity. Methods need to be revalidated on a regular basis to ensure they are suitable to analyze materials in use at that point of time. Any change in equipment or instrumentation or premises may also call for a revalidation of the analytical method.

Steps in Analytical Method Validation

1. Planning analytical method validation.
2. Writing the protocol and getting it approved.
3. Executing the approved protocol.
4. Analyzing validation data obtained.
5. Reporting results of validation.
6. Finalizing the analytical method procedure based on validation results.

Contents of Analytical Method Validation Protocol

1. Objective.
2. Parameters to be evaluated.
3. Acceptance criteria for above parameters.
4. Experiment details.
5. Analytical procedure in draft form.
6. Procedure to deal with errors/deviations.
7. Methods to be used for data analysis.

14.3.8.2 Analytical Method Validation Parameters/ Characteristics

The analytical performance parameters that must be a part of validation programs include the following:

- Accuracy
- Precision

- Specificity
- Detection limit
- Quantitation limit
- Linearity
- Range robustness

14.3.8.2.1 Accuracy

The International Convention on Harmonization (ICH) definition of states that "Accuracy of an analytical procedure is the closeness of agreement between the values that are accepted either as conventional true values or an accepted reference value and the value found.

For a drug substance, accuracy is determined by applying the analytical method to an analyte whose purity is known, such as a reference standard.

For drug products, accuracy is determined by applying the analytical method to mixtures containing drug components along with a known amount of analyte that has been added, within the operating range of the method.

According to ICH guidelines, a minimum of nine determinations must be performed over a minimum of three concentration levels that cover the specified range.

Accuracy is generally reported in terms of percent recovery (by the assay) of the known amount of analyte added into the sample. It may also be reported in terms of the difference between accepted true value and the mean, along with the confidence intervals.

Generally, accuracy of recovery for drug substances must be between 99 – 101%. For drug product, the values may range between 98 – 102%. Any accuracy of recovery data that deviates from this range must be investigated in detail.

14.3.8.2.2 Precision

Precision is defined as the degree of closeness of a series of measurements obtained using multiple samples of the same substance under specified conditions.

Precision may be studied as three characteristics – repeatability, intermediate precision and reproducibility.

Repeatability measures precision under same conditions over short time duration. This is done using normal operating conditions and same equipment as usually used for the given analytical method. ICH guidelines prescribe that at least nine determinations should be run over the range specified for the procedure. Values to be reported include standard devition, coefficient of variation (relative standard deviation) and confidence interval.

Intermediate precision refers to variation occurring within the same testing laboratory. It includes a study of day-to-day variation, equipment variation and analyst variation.

Reproducibility gives information about precision of measurements between laboratories. To validate reproducibility, the same study must be performed using same experimental design and same sample lot at the different laboratories.

14.3.8.2.3 Specificity

ICH definition of specificity is "The ability to assess unequivocally, an analyte, in the presence of other components that are expected to be present".

A test method is called specific if it is able to discriminate the compound of interest from other closely related compounds that may be present in the same sample. Samples containing the analyte must show positive result; samples without the analyte must show negative result. Also, when closely related compounds are tested, the test method must not show positive result.

14.3.8.2.4 Detection Limit

Detection limit (DL) is defined as the "lowest amount of analyte present in a sample that can be detected but not necessarily quantitated under the stated experimental conditions." DL is generally expressed in terms of analyte concentraton in the sample (as parts per million, or percentage). DL may be established visually, or using signal-to-noise ratios, or using data from standard deviation and slope of calibration curve.

14.3.8.2.5 Quantitation Limit

Quantitation limit (QL) is defined as the lowest level of an analyte that can be quantitatively measured under the given experimental conditions. This parameter is generally useful to assay analytes present in very low levels – for example, degradation products or impurities. QL may also be defined as concentration of a related substance in the sample that produces a signal-to-noise ratio of 10 : 1. QL for a method is influenced by two important factors – the accuracy in sample preparation and sensitivity of the detector used.

QL may be evaluated by visual method, signal-to-noise ratio method and the calibration curve method. Once QL has been determined, it must be further validated by carrying out accuracy and precision measurements at this level.

14.3.8.2.6 Linearity

As per ICH guidelines, linearity is defined as, "The ability (within a particular range) to obtain test results of variable data (such as area under the curve, or absorbance) which are directly proportional to the concentration of the analyte in the sample. Analyte quantitation may be done using variables such as peak height, peak area or ratio of peak heights/areas of analyte to internal standard.

Linearity may be determined by two methods. The first one involves directly weighing different quantities of standard to prepare solutions of different concentrations. The second and more popular approach is to prepare high concentration stock solutions and then dilute it to lower concentrations.

Linearity is accepted if the coefficient of determination is found to be greater than or equal to 0.997. ICH guidelines required reporting of slope, y-intercept and residual sum of squares, too.

14.3.8.2.7 Range

Range is defined as the interval between lower and upper concentrations of analyte in the sample for analytical procedure that is demonstrated to possess a suitable level of accuracy, precision and linearity. Assays must generally have a range of 80 – 120% of nominal concentration. Content uniformity tests must have range of 70 – 130% of the nominal concentration.

14.3.8.2.8 Robustness

It is defined as the capability of an analytical method to remain unaffected by small but deliberate variations in the method parameters. This characteristic indicates how reliable a given analytical method is during normal usage conditions.

14.3.8.3 Finalizing the Analytical Procedure

Following a successful analytical method validation, the final analytical procedure must be established and documented. The minimum information to be provided in this document includes:

1. Rationale for the procedure and capabilities of the method. If the method is a revised one, advantages of the revision must be described.
2. Complete details of analytical procedure to allow the method to be replicated by anyone reading it. All important instructions and parameters must be mentioned here, along with formulae for calculation of results.
3. List of impurities that are permitted, and their limits for impurity assays.
4. Validate data.
5. Revision history.
6. Signatures of authorized personnel (author of the procedure, reviewer, management and QA representatives).

14.3.8.4 Analytical Method Revalidation

Validated methods need to be revalidated in the following situations:

1. When a significant change has been introduced in the process of synthesizing the drug substance (API).
2. When a new impurity is encountered, changing the specificity profile of the method.
3. If changes are made in excipient composition which can introduce new impurities.
4. When there is change in major equipment or change of API supplier that may change degradation profile of the API.

Validation is one of the most important concepts in the area of drug development and manufacturing. By promising consistent and reliable processes, validation helps to ensure products are manufactured with desired quality attributes each and every time a process is run. Thus, it plays a crucial role in achieving the objective of QA that quality will be designed and built into the product instead of being merely tested at the final stages.

Calibration of pH meter:

This uses the two-point calibration method which is performed using two buffers of known pH. One of them is a pH 7.0 standard buffer and the other is either an acidic or alkaline buffer of known pH. It is important to make sure that all buffers are at the same temperature before beginning the calibration because pH often varies with temperature.

1. Switch on the pH meter, and wait for enough time for it to warm up (as per information in the instrument's operating manual).

2. Remove the electrode from its storage solution, rinse with distilled water and blot dry using a piece of tissue paper. Avoid rubbing the electrode while drying to prevent damage to the sensitive membrane that surrounds it.

3. Place the electrode tip into buffer solution of pH 7.00 and press the "Measure" or "Calibrate" button, and wait for the display to stabilize.

4. Adjust the calibration button to make the display read 7 if required.

5. Remove the electrode from the buffer solution, rinse with distilled water and blot dry using fresh tissue paper.

6. Place the electrode into buffer solution of either pH 4.01 or pH 9.20 and wait for the display to stabilize.

7. Adjust the calibration button to make the display read the pH as 4.01 or 9.20 depending on which buffer you have used.

8. Remove the electrode from the buffer, clean with distilled water, and blot dry with tissue paper.

9. Place the dried electrode back into the storage solution.

Qualification of UV-Visible Spectrophotometer:

The UV-Visible spectrophotometer is an instrument that is used to measure absorbance of solutions over the ultraviolet and visible ranges of the electromagnetic spectrum, generally between 200 – 800 nanometres.

Qualification may be defined as the act of proving and documenting that a given equipment or process or utility is correctly installed, working properly, and is consistently producing the expected results.

Qualification of the UV-Visible spectrophotometer involves the following steps:

1. **Design qualification:** The type and make of the instrument to be purchased must be chosen carefully depending on the specific requirements of the type of samples that will need to be measured.

2. **Installation qualification:**

   (a) Install the instrument in a room that is maintained at temperature between 15 - 25°C and relative humidity of 45 – 80%.

   (b) The installation site must be away from dust, corrosive liquids or gases and direct sunlight.

   (c) Remove the instrument from its packing material, and place it on a surface that does not vibrate.

   (d) Install the computer near the instrument, or load the software into an existing computer.

(d) Check the following parameters at this stage:

Parameters	Specification
Appearance	Intact, no defects visible
Operational manual provided	Must be present
Parts	All parts present as per operating manual
Hardware and software supplied	Must be present

3. Operational qualification:

(a) Connect the instrument to the mains and switch it on.

(b) Follow the operating manual instructions and check for the following parameters: Wavelength accuracy, linearity of absorbance, resolution, wavelength reproducibility, photometric accuracy, stray light, photometric noise, baseline flatness and photometric stability.

(c) Measure the values obtained for each of the above parameters and check if they meet the specified acceptance criteria. Record these values.

4. Performance qualification:

(a) Define the performance criteria that are most important to routine operations.

(b) Define the acceptance criteria for these performance criteria selected.

(c) Determine the values for the chosen criteria and check if they meet the acceptance limits set.

(d) Decide on the frequency of regular calibration and performance qualification for routine use of the instrument.

REVIEW QUESTIONS

1. Define calibration and write a note on its significance.
2. How frequently must equipment be calibrated?
3. Discuss the different phases of qualification of equipment.
4. What is a Validation Master Plan? Which are its important elements?
5. Define analytical method validation.
6. Define the terms accuracy, precision and specificity.
7. What are detection limit and quantitation limit? Differentiate between them.
8. Explain linearity and range of a method.

Chapter ... 15

GOOD WAREHOUSING PRACTICE AND MATERIALS MANAGEMENT

Objectives:

Upon completion of this section, the student should be able to

- Explain requirements of good warehousing practices.
- Describe segregation of materials stored in a warehouse.
- Outline the procedures in receiving, handling and storing materials in a warehouse.
- List and explain the records to be maintained in a pharmaceutical warehouse.
- Describe stock management in the warehouse.
- Explain role of the warehouse in product recall.

Introduction

In the pharmaceutical industry, it is critical to pay attention to the storage and distribution of products. Medicines need to be stored under very specific conditions to ensure they retain their quality. Different dosage forms must be stored and transported under different environmental conditions and therefore, there cannot be one general rule for their handling. Thus, it is vital to follow good warehousing practices and good distribution practices to ensure the quality of products is maintained.

The WHO guide to good storage practices for pharmaceuticals highlights the following important areas for the warehousing of pharmaceuticals.

15.1 PERSONNEL

All sites where pharmaceutical products are stored (manufacturing unit, distributor /wholesaler /retail sale pharmacy premises) must have a sufficient number of appropriately qualified and trained personnel. The staff must be given the necessary training on good storage practices, the best practices to adopt, and safety issues. They must also be trained on matters of personal hygiene, good sanitation practices, use of working garments and suitable protective clothing. Those employees who work in special storage areas (such as cold stores, for example) must be trained on the regulations and procedures particular to their work.

15.2 PREMISES AND FACILITIES

15.2.1 Storage areas

1. **Entry:** Entry into storage areas must be controlled, and only authorized persons must be permitted to enter.

2. **Size:** The areas must be of a size sufficient to allow the systematic storage of different categories of materials such as raw materials, packaging materials, intermediate products, bulk products and finished products. There must be separate areas for products in quarantine, approved products and products that have been rejected, returned or recalled from the market.

3. **Storage conditions:** The storage areas must be designed to allow optimum storage conditions. They must be dry and clean at all times. Temperature and relative humidity must be maintained within the prescribed limits. There must be provisions to check, monitor and record these parameters. All materials must be stored off the floor on racks or pallets, with sufficient space in between to permit easy cleaning as well as inspection if required. The pallets and racks must be kept clean and well-maintained.

4. **Cleanliness:** The storage areas should be cleaned regularly to avoid the accumulation of waste. Measures should be taken to prevent the entry of vermin. There must be written instructions available that indicate the cleaning methods to be adopted and the frequency of cleaning. Systems must be set up for pest control and written instructions provided. Agents used for pest control must be safe, and not cause any contamination of the materials being stored. Adequate measures must be taken to clean any product spillage, in order to avoid the risk of contaminating other products in the storage area.

5. **External areas:** Receiving and dispatch areas in the warehouse should be designed to protect materials from weather conditions. The design of receiving areas should be such as to allow cleaning of incoming materials before storage, if necessary.

6. Quarantine areas – Areas meant for storage of products in quarantine must be clearly indicated, and be situated separate from the general storage areas. Entry into this area must be restricted to only those personnel who are authorized. Non-physical quarantine methods may be used (computerized systems, for example) provided they are validated to prove they provide a secure system equivalent to that of a physical quarantine.

7. **Sampling:** Separate sampling area for starting materials must be provided in a controlled environment. When sampling is done in the storage area itself, care must be taken to prevent contamination of other products or cross-contamination. This area must be regularly cleaned.

8. **Storage of rejected, expired, returned or recalled materials or products:** Separate areas must be provided for storing rejected, expired, returned or recalled materials or products. Such materials must be conspicuously market to avoid inadvertent mix-ups. Physical segregation is best; non-physical systems (electronic) must be validated to prove they provide adequate levels of security.

9. **Special materials storage:** Pharmaceutical products that are sensitive, dangerous, hazardous, narcotic, radioactive and/or highly active as well as substances with a risk of fire, explosion or abuse must be stored in dedicated areas with sufficient security and safety measures in place.

10. **Handling and distribution:** All materials in the storage area must be handled, stored and distributed in keeping with GMP guidelines. Procedures must be designed to prevent mix-ups, contamination and cross-contamination. Storage conditions should ensure quality is maintained at all times.

11. **Rotation of stock:** All stocks in the warehouse must be rotated appropriately, following the "First Expired/First Out (FEFO)" principles.

12. **Rejected materials:** Products and materials that have been rejected must be clearly marked and controlled with a quarantine system that prevents their use until their fate is decided.

13. **Narcotic drugs storage:** Storage of narcotic drugs must comply with international conventions as well as national laws regarding narcotic storage.

14. **Damaged items:** Damaged and broken items must be immediately removed from the usable stock and stored separately until their fate is decided.

15. **Lighting:** Storage areas must be lighted appropriately to allow the safe and accurate performance of all operations in the warehouse.

15.2.2 Storage Conditions

All pharmaceutical materials and products must be stored in compliance with the requirements specified on the respective labels. These specifications must be based on the results obtained during the stability testing of the respective products. Storage conditions must be regularly monitored to ensure compliance with requirements. Recorded data (temperature, relative humidity etc.) must be available if required for review. Data monitoring and recording equipment must be checked and calibrated at predetermined intervals; results of these checks must be recorded and maintained for a duration of shelf life of the product plus one year, or as specified in the national regulations. Monitoring equipment must be located in those areas which are most likely to experience fluctuations; this equipment must be regularly calibrated.

15.3 STORAGE REQUIREMENTS

15.3.1 Documentation

1. **Instructions and records:** Written instructions as well as records must be available to document all activities taking place in the storage area, including those related to expired stock handling. The route taken by the products and information through the organization in case of product recall must be described in sufficient detail.

2. **Information of each product:** Each material or product stored must have permanent information (in either written or electronic form) to provide information regarding the storage conditions, precautions if any to be observed, and dates for re-test. Labels must be in keeping with requirements as per the respective pharmacopoeias and current national regulations.

3. **Delivery records:** Records must be maintained for every delivery, and must include information regarding description of the goods, quantity, quality, supplier and the batch number, receipt date, assigned batch number and expiry date. These records must be retained for a duration equal to shelf life of the goods plus one year or as specified in the national regulations.

4. **Comprehensive records:** All details regarding the materials and pharmaceutical products received and issued in the warehouse must be recorded and maintained by a specific system to permit their identification such as by batch number.

15.3.2 Labelling and Containers

1. **Storage containers:** Pharmaceutical products and all materials must be stored in appropriate containers so that their quality is not affected. The containers must provide sufficient protection from external factors such as bacterial contamination.

2. **Container labeling:** The minimum labeling requirements for containers include details of – name of the material with pharmacopoeial reference where applicable (proper name only, no code names or abbreviations can be used without authorization), batch number, expiry date, re-test date and storage conditions to be maintained.

15.3.3 Receiving Incoming Materials

1. **Verification:** Every incoming delivery must be checked immediately against the details given in the purchase order. All containers must be physically verified by description on the label, type of material, batch number and quantity.

2. **Uniformity:** The uniformity of the containers must be verified. Further subdivision may be done in keeping with the supplier's batch number in cases where the delivery contains more than a single batch of product.

3. **Inspection:** Every container must be carefully checked for any contamination, damage or tampering. If the inspection reveals evidence of such incident, the entire consignment must be kept under quarantine until further investigation.

4. **Sampling:** Sampling should be done only by authorized personnel who are adequately qualified and trained, in keeping with written instructions for sampling. Labels must be affixed on the containers from which samples have been drawn.

5. **Quarantine:** Goods must be stored under quarantine after sampling until authorized release or rejection instructions are obtained. Separate batches must be stored segregated from each other.

6. **Rejected materials:** Rejected materials must be stored segregated from other products to prevent their accidental use. Appropriate measures must be taken to either return them to the supplier or to destroy them if deemed necessary.

Warning signs of problems with incoming materials:

1. **Odors:** May indicate spillage of product. In some cases, may indicate interactions of cleaning agent/preservative with drug product.

2. **Moisture/fluid:** Evidence of damage in packaging that has caused drug to leak. May also warn of premises being exposed to moisture/the elements.

3. **Spillage:** Medicines loose from their original container indicate damage to package. In some cases, it renders the product unsafe and unfit for use.

4. **Dirt, tears, scratches, animal feces:** Indicate activity of pests such as rodents which have used the shipping material for shelter. Safety of the drugs may be compromised because these pests may carry diseases too.

5. **Damaged/tampered temperature tags:** Tags are used to record temperature conditions under which shipping was done for thermolabile products. Damaged/tampererd tags indicate deviations from required temperature, which may have rendered the product unsafe for use.

15.3.4 Stock Rotation and Control

Periodically, the actual stock in the warehouse must be compared with the recorded quantity of stocks. If such reconciliation reveals discrepancies, they must be investigated to find out if material has been incorrectly issued or if there has been a mix-up. Containers that have been partly used must be closed and sealed securely to prevent contamination and spoilage. Previously opened or partly used containers must be used up before fresh containers are opened. Containers that have been damaged must not be issued unless tests have shown that the quality of the product is unaffected by the damage.

15.3.5 Control of Obsolete and Outdated Products

Stock in the warehouse must be periodically checked and expired/obsolete/outdated products and materials must be removed. Until such material is removed, precautions must be taken to ensure they are not issued for use.

15.4 RETURNED GOODS

Goods whether returned or recalled from the market, must be handled according to approved procedures. Records of the same should be maintained. All such goods must be kept in quarantine until a decision has been taken by the nominated, responsible person. Goods that pass a quality re-evaluation may be returned to stock approved for sale. Records of such events must be maintained in the stock records. Any pharmaceutical product returned by patients to the pharmacy must be destroyed.

15.5 DISPATCH AND TRANSPORTATION OF GOODS

The dispatch and transport of pharmaceutical products must be done under conditions that ensure the prescribed storage conditions are maintained, and integrity of the product is not affected. When dry ice is used, care must be taken to ensure it does not come into contact with the product as it may cause freezing of the product. When material is being transported, devices must be used to monitor temperature conditions; records of such monitoring must be maintained.

Any transportation must proceed only on receiving a delivery order. Documents must be maintained showing the delivery order and dispatch details. External containers must be clearly labeled in indelible ink, and must provide adequate protection to the product from weather conditions. Dispatch records must contain the following details at the very minimum – dispatch date, customer name and address, product description (name, strength, dosage form), quantity, batch number, storage conditions.

15.6 PRODUCT RECALL

Appropriate procedures must be set in place for the prompt and effective market recalls of known or suspected defective product. Product recalls may be triggered by any of the following situations:

- Customer complaints that draw attention to a critical quality defect.
- Reports of adverse drug reactions.
- Samples retained for stability studies show deterioration of product quality.
- GMP deviations uncovered during regulatory inspections.
- Information becomes available indicating that counterfeit or tampered product has been supplied in place of authentic drug.

Case Study of Tylenol

In 2010, McNeil Consumer Healthcare, a division of Johnson and Johnson, announced a recall of extra strength Tylenol, Tylenol grape meltaway tablets, Tylenol rapid release gel caps and some other products due to complaints of a musty, moldy smell and black particles. Similar complaints had been received even in 2008 and 2009, leading to recall of some lots of their products. Some patients complained of not just the smell but also nausea, vomiting, stomach pain and diarrhea. Post these events, an investigation was conducted by the company, and the results showed the odour to be caused due to traces of a chemical named 2,4,6-tribromoanisole (TBA). This chemical was used as a preservative on wooden pallets that were employed in the storing and transporting of the Tylenol product plastic bottles.

Once finished products reach the warehouse, they are not subjected to any further testing or inspection. If products undergo deterioration or damage at this stage, it may go unnoticed, and a harmful product may find its way to the patient. It is therefore vital that good warehousing practices must be followed by adequately trained personnel to make sure that the quality of the product reaching the end user is the same as it was when it left the manufacturing unit.

REVIEW QUESTIONS

1. Discuss the requirements of good warehousing practices.
2. Explain the steps in receiving and storage of materials in the warehouse.
3. Enumerate the precautions to be taken when handling goods in the warehouse.
4. List and describe the records to be maintained in a pharmaceutical warehouse.
5. Explain the stock rotation principle used in pharmaceutical storage.
6. Discuss the segregation of materials in a warehouse.

✍ ✍ ✍

REFERENCES

References

1. World Health Organization. (2007). Quality Assurance of Pharmaceuticals: A Compendium of Guidelines and Related Materials. Vol 2, 2nd Updated Edition. Good Manufacturing Practices and Inspection. Available online at https://www.who.int/medicines/areas/quality_safety/quality_assurance/QualityAssurancePharmVol2.pdf

2. Potdar M.A. (2007). Pharmaceutical Quality Assurance. 2nd Edition. Nirali Prakashan.

3. Sharma P. P. (2015). How to Practice GMPs: A Treatise on GMPs. 7th Edition. Vandana Publications.

4. Ministry of Health and Family Welfare, India. Schedule M: Drugs and Cosmetics Rules, 1945. Available online at https://ipapharma.org/wp-content/uploads/2019/02/schedule-m-1.pdf

5. United States Food and Drug Administration. 21 CFR Part 211. Available online at https://www.accessdata.fda.gov/scripts/cdrh/cfdocs/cfcfr/CFRSearch.cfm?CFRPart= 211

6. Rahalkar H (2012) Historical Overview of Pharmaceutical Industry and Drug Regulatory Affairs. Pharmaceut Reg Affairs S11:002. doi:10.4172/2167-7689. S11-002. Available online at https://www.omicsonline.org/open-access/historical-overview-of-pharmaceutical-industry-and-drug-regulatory-affairs-2167-7689.S11-002.pdf

7. ICH Official Website. Available online at https://www.ich.org/

8. Schlindwein W.S. and Gibson M. (2018). Pharmaceutical Quality by Design: A Practical Approach. John Wiley and Sons Ltd.

9. Chakravarty, A., Parmar, N. K., & Ranyal, R. K. (2001). Total Quality Management - The New Paradigm in Health Care Management. Medical journal, Armed Forces India, 57(3), 226–229. doi:10.1016/S0377-1237(01)80049-6 Available online at https://www.ncbi.nlm.nih.gov/pmc/articles/PMC4925033/

10. Bhavya K, Manisha Vishnumurthy K, Rambabu D and Sumakanth M. (2019). ICH guidelines – "Q" series (quality guidelines) - A review. GSC Biological and Pharmaceutical Sciences, 6(3), 89-106. Available online at https://gsconlinepress.com/journals/gscbps/sites/default/files/GSCBPS-2019-0034.pdf

11. Yu, L. X., Amidon, G., Khan, M. A., Hoag, S. W., Polli, J., Raju, G. K., & Woodcock, J. (2014). Understanding pharmaceutical quality by design. *The AAPS journal*, *16*(4), 771–783. doi:10.1208/s12248-014-9598-3 Available online at https://www.ncbi.nlm.nih.gov/pmc/articles/PMC4070262/

12. Food and Drug Administration (FDA) (2004). Guidance for Industry: PAT – A Framework for Innovative Pharmaceutical Development, Manufacturing, and Quality Assurance.

13. Vemuri P. K. and Gupta N. V. (2015). A Review on Quality by Design Approach for Pharmaceuticals. Int. Jour of Drug Dev & Res. Available online at http://www.ijddr.in/drug-development/a-review-on-quality-by-design-approach-qbd-for-pharmaceuticals.php?aid=5482

14. Ausin C. (2018). A Regulatory Perspective on the Use of Prior Knowledge. Available online at https://cdn.ymaws.com/www.casss.org/resource/resmgr/cmc_no_am_jan_spkr_slds/2018_WCBP_AusinCristina.pdf

15. International Organization for Standardization website. Available online at https://www.iso.org/home.html

16. Handoo A and Sood S. K. (2012). Clinical Laboratory Accreditation in India. Clin Lab Med. doi: 10.1016/j.cll.2012.04.009. Available online at https://www.ncbi.nlm.nih.gov/pubmed/22727005

17. Panadda S. (2007). WHO: Guidelines for Establishment of Accreditation of Health Laboratories. Available online at http://apps.searo.who.int/PDS_DOCS/B3179.pdf

18. Website of National Accreditation Board for Testing and Calibration Laboratories available online at https://nabl-india.org/faq/

19. Kanagasabapathy A.S. and Rao P. (2005). Laboratory Accreditation – Procedural Guidelines. Ind Jour of Clin Biochem. Available online at http://medind.nic.in/iaf/t05/i2/iaft05i2p186.pdf

20. Ministry of Health and Family Welfare, India. Schedule M: Drugs and Cosmetics Rules, 1945. Available online at https://ipapharma.org/wp-content/uploads/2019/02/schedule-m-1.pdf

21. United States Food and Drug Administration. 21 CFR Part 211. Available online at https://www.accessdata.fda.gov/scripts/cdrh/cfdocs/cfcfr/CFRSearch.cfm?CFRPart=211&showFR=1&subpartNode=21:4.0.1.1.11.2

22. World Health Organization. (2011). Technical Report Series No. 961, Annex 3: WHO Good Manufacturing Practices for Pharmaceutical Products: Main Principles. Available online at https://www.who.int/medicines/areas/quality_safety/quality_assurance/GMPPharmaceuticalProductsMainPrinciplesTRS961Annex3.pdf

23. World Health Organization. (2014). WHO Technical Report Series No. 986. Annex 2: WHO Good Manufacturing Practices for Pharmaceutical Products: Main Principles. Available online at http://apps.who.int/medicinedocs/documents/s21467en/s21467en.pdf

24. Government of India, Ministry of Health. (2014). Pharmacopoeia of India. Volume II. Controller of Publications

25. Dean D.A, Evans E.R., and Hall I.H. (2000). Pharmaceutical Packaging Technology. Taylor & Francis. Available online at https://farmacotecnia2015.files.wordpress.com/2015/05/pharmaceutical-packaging-technology.pdf

26. USFDA Center for Drug Evaluation and Research. (2006). Guidance for Industry Investigating Out-of-Specification (OOS) Test Results for Pharmaceutical Production. Available online at https://www.fda.gov/media/71001/download

27. United States Food and Drug Administration. Part 58 Good Laboratory Practice for Non-clinical Laboratory Studies. Available online at https://www.accessdata.fda.gov/scripts/cdrh/cfdocs/cfcfr/CFRSearch.cfm?CFRPart=58

28. Baldeshwiler A.M. (2003). History of FDA Good Laboratory Practices. 2003 John Wiley & Sons, Ltd. Qual Assur J 2003; 7, 157–161. DOI: 10.1002/qaj.228 Available online at https://onlinelibrary.wiley.com/doi/pdf/10.1002/qaj.228

29. Central Drugs Standard Control Organisation (2017). Guidelines on Recall and Rapid Alert System for Drugs (Including Biologicals & Vaccines). Available online at https://cdsco.gov.in/opencms/export/sites/CDSCO_WEB/Pdf-documents/biologicals/4GuidelineRecalRapidAlert.pdf

30. World Health Organization (1999). Guidelines for Safe Disposal of Unwanted Pharmaceuticals in and after Emergencies. Available online at https://www.who.int/water_sanitation_health/medicalwaste/unwantpharm.pdf

31. Nagaich, U., & Sadhna, D. (2015). Drug recall: An incubus for pharmaceutical companies and most serious drug recall of history. International journal of pharmaceutical investigation, 5(1), 13–19. doi:10.4103/2230-973X.147222 Available online at https://www.ncbi.nlm.nih.gov/pmc/articles/PMC4286830/

32. Sreekanth K, Gupta V. N., Raghunanda H.V. and Nitin K.U. A Review on Managing of Pharmaceutical Waste in Industry. International Journal of PharmTech Research. 2014; 6(3):899-907. Available online at https://www.researchgate.net/publication/263657517_A_Review_on_Managing_of_Pharmaceutical_Waste_in_Industry

33. Jaseem M., Kumar P. and Remya M.J. An overview of waste management in pharmaceutical industry. The Pharma Innovation Journal 2017; 6(3): 158-161. Available online at http://www.thepharmajournal.com/archives/2017/vol6issue3/PartC/6-2-9-174.pdf

34. Indian Pharmaceutical Alliance. (2018). Good Documentation Practice (GDP) Guideline. Available online at https://www.ipa-india.org/static-files/pdf/event/ipf2018-presentation22.pdf

35. World Health Organization (2016). WHO Technical Report Series No. 996. Annex 5: Guidance on good data and record management practices. Available online at https://www.who.int/medicines/publications/pharmprep/WHO_TRS_996_annex05.pdf

36. Patel, K., & Chotai, N. (2011). Documentation and Records: Harmonized GMP Requirements. *Journal of young pharmacists : JYP*, *3*(2), 138–150. doi:10.4103/0975-1483.80303. Available online at https://www.ncbi.nlm.nih.gov/pmc/articles/PMC3122044/#CIT11

37. Gad S.C. (2008) Pharmaceutical Manufacturing Handbook: Regulations and Quality. John Wiley & Sons, Inc. Available online at https://gmpua.com/Process/RegulationsAndQuality.pdf

38. Keyur B.A., Singh K.D et al. (2014). Overview of Validation and Basic Concepts of Process Validation. Sch. Acad. J. Pharm.; 3(2): 178-190 Available online at https://pdfs.semanticscholar.org/974b/f78fed920857276ceaff39948d24a36fb00e.pdf

39. World Health Organization. (1996). WHO Expert Committee on Specifications for Pharmaceutical Preparations - WHO Technical Report Series, No. 863 - Thirty-fourth Report. Available online at https://apps.who.int/medicinedocs/en/d/Js5516e/

40. World Health Organization Technical Report Series No. 908, Annex 9. (2003). Guide to good storage practices for pharmaceuticals. Available online at:
https://apps.who.int/medicinedocs/documents/s18675en/s18675en.pdf

41. Organization of Pharmaceutical Producers of India. (2014). Guidelines on Good Distribution Practices for Pharmaceutical Products. Available online at:
https://www.indiaoppi.com/sites/default/files/PDF%20files/OPPI%20book%20Guidelines%20on%20Good%20Distribution%20Practices%20%28final%29.pdf

42. World Health Organization Technical Report Series No. 957, Annex 5. (2010). WHO Good Distribution Practices for Pharmaceutical Products. Available online at:
https://www.who.int/medicines/areas/quality_safety/quality_assurance/GoodDistributionPracticesTRS957Annex5.pdf

✍ ✍ ✍